healthy nutrition

World Health Organization
Regional Office for Europe
Copenhagen

Healthy nutrition

Preventing nutrition-related diseases in Europe

W.P.T. James

in collaboration with
A. Ferro-Luzzi, B. Isaksson
and W.B. Szostak

WHO Regional Publications, European Series, No. 24

ICP/NUT 114/s02
Text editing by: M.S. Burgher
Cover photo by: Anna Ferro-Luzzi
           Taken in a village south of Rome

ISBN 92 890 1115 7
ISSN 0378-2255

PRINTED IN DENMARK

CONTENTS

Acknowledgements

We are indebted to a great number of experts who have given their time to help prepare this book. Their documents have been used freely. Particular mention should be made of the help obtained from Dr Z.J. Brzeziński, and from the staff of the Epidemiology and Statistics unit of the WHO Regional Office for Europe. We are also grateful to Dr C. Muir of the International Agency for Research on Cancer (IARC), to participants in the countrywide integrated noncommunicable diseases intervention (CINDI) programme, and to those involved in the project on European risk factors and incidence — a collaborative analysis (ERICA) for making data available. Professor L. Hallberg kindly provided help with the section on iron-deficiency anaemia. A great deal of work in the preparation of this report has come from Mrs Jean James and from the Nutrition unit in the WHO Regional Office for Europe.

Foreword

Patterns of disease in Europe are changing; statistics prove it. Patterns of diet are changing as well, as are other aspects of lifestyle. People are often unaware of how much their eating patterns have actually changed, and surprised when confronted with the evidence. Put in simple terms, people can now eat every day the foods that our ancestors had only on festive occasions. And, as our forebears have told us, too much feasting is not good for health.

This book describes in detail how dietary patterns have evolved in Europe, how patterns of disease have changed, and what the nature of the relationship between these developments might be.

The new food situation in Europe, with enough to eat for everybody, with famine and starvation seemingly only a remote possibility, and with overproduction the predominant problem in agriculture, presents us with an entirely new set of problems.

The question of food production in Europe today really concerns not quantity but quality. The planning of a population's food supply must eventually include not only aspects of economy and policies on farming and food manufacture, but also health aspects. In short, there is now a case for making nutrition policies rather than food policies only.

This is a challenge to nutritionists: to expand their skills so that they can convey their knowledge about the effects of nutrients on human physiology to those who produce and process these nutrients. This transfer of knowledge, however, is only the first of their new tasks. Nutritionists have to get out of their laboratories and be ready to discuss foods on a national as well as a personal level. Alternative strategies for producing and processing food have to be formulated and discussed. The nutritionist looking at the overall picture has an important role in translating the findings of food and nutritional science and nutritional epidemiology into approaches relevant to the consumer. Action to help change people's eating habits in desired directions will also be needed.

It is imperative, then, to know what these desired directions actually are. In other words, the aims and objectives of a nutrition policy should be very clearly spelled out at the outset of policy formulation.

The process of making nutrition policies can be lengthy and complicated, but it will eventually be possible to evaluate the effects of such a policy on food consumption patterns at regular intervals — for example, annually. Setting objectives is essential for the evaluation process.

A nutrition policy leads to the establishment of objectives, and it is necessary to spell out exactly what the consequences of its adoption will be. Makers of policy on the food and agriculture industries will use these objectives in their planning. To help them in their task the Regional Officer for Nutrition in the WHO Regional Office for Europe asked Professors James, Ferro-Luzzi, Isaksson and Szostak to write this book. Their first draft was circulated in the summer of 1986. Special mention should be made of Elisabet Helsing, Regional Officer for Nutrition, who through her drive and initiative has created the WHO nutrition programme for Europe. It is thanks to her organizing ability and vision that this framework for a nutrition policy for Europe has been developed.

The enthusiastic reception of the first draft by nutritionists all over Europe demonstrated the need for international documentation of the relationship between diet and health. As an increasing number of countries move towards formulating food health policies, it is hoped that this book will be instrumental in the setting of objectives.

As national committees revise their recommendations on nutrient intakes, this book will also require revision, to reflect advances in nutritional knowledge. Nutrition is a science in a dynamic phase of development. This dynamism must be reflected in nutrition policy-making, as well.

A nutrition policy must also be seen in a wider context, as forming a part of the overall health policy of a country (in the same way that the European health for all policy and its 38 targets fit into health policy). To promote healthy eating habits, a nutrition policy outlines the need for national policies and programmes to ensure: that policies on agriculture and food production aim at the wide availability of healthy food; that policies on the pricing, advertising, and preparation and sale of food make healthy food attractive to the consumer; and that educational policy motivates people to buy healthy food and to adopt healthy eating habits. Such a development will have a very positive effect on the health of Europeans.

This book is a clear challenge to all governments; to European farmers; to the European food processing industry; to restaurants, cafeterias, and fast-food chains; to health personnel, teachers, dietitians and cooks; and, ultimately, for anyone among Europe's 850 million people cooking a meal!

J.E. Asvall
*WHO Regional Director
for Europe*

Executive summary

In 1982 a WHO expert committee developed a set of nutrient goals that was considered optimal for the prevention of coronary heart disease in a population. These goals, which specify the amounts of nutrients that people need, were established as average intakes for the whole population, additional recommendations being made for people at high risk of heart disease.

The present publication sets out information on the prevalence of a number of nutrition-related diseases in Europe and considers the available data on dietary patterns and nutrient intakes. A brief analysis is also made of the basis for thinking that diet plays a role in the development of these diseases. In Europe as a whole, about half the premature deaths in men and women below the age of 65 years result from diseases to which diet makes an important contribution. Coronary heart disease, stroke, many kinds of cancer, oral disease, anaemia, goitre, cirrhosis of the liver, diabetes, gallstones, obesity, high blood pressure and bone disease in the elderly have a huge effect on medical services. These conditions should be considered preventable, even if the precise way in which dietary deficiencies or excesses lead to them remains obscure. An analysis of the dietary factors involved suggests that a common set of nutrient goals can be developed as desirable national health goals for the people of Europe.

The following table summarizes most of these nutrient goals. Others follow the table. They have been collated from the recommendations of various national committees and are based mainly on what is widely considered to be an ideal nutritional pattern for the prevention of non-communicable diseases. The greater precision in the definition of nutrient goals presented here in comparison to those advocated in 1982 by the WHO Expert Committee on the Prevention of Coronary Heart Disease simply ensures conformity with the intermediate goals advocated by national and other WHO committees. It is clear that the recommendations of national committees are similar, although the nutrient patterns of the countries concerned differ markedly from the goals. These national recommendations can therefore be seen as pragmatic objectives that aim to move the nutritional pattern of a country towards the ideal nutrient goals. The intermediate goals may be particularly appropriate for northern European countries. Existing national European nutrition policies also relate to the whole

Table 1. Intermediate and ultimate nutrient goals for Europe

	Intermediate goals		Ultimate goals
	General population	Cardiovascular high-risk group	
Percentage of total energy[a] derived from:			
complex carbohydrates[b]	>40	>45	45–55
protein	12–13	12–13	12–13
sugar	10	10	10
total fat	35	30	20–30
saturated fat	15	10	10
P:S ratio[c]	≦0.5	≦1.0	≦1.0
Dietary fibre (g/day)[d]	30	>30	>30
Salt (g/day)	7–8	5	5
Cholesterol (mg/4.18 MJ)	—	<100	<100
Water fluoride (mg/litre)	0.7–1.2	0.7–1.2	0.7–1.2

[a] All the values given refer to alcohol-free total energy intakes.

[b] The complex carbohydrate figures are implications of the other recommendations.

[c] This is the ratio of polyunsaturated to saturated fatty acids.

[d] Dietary fibre values are based on analytical methods that measure non-starch polysaccharide and the enzyme-resistant starch produced by food processing or cooking methods.

The following are both ultimate nutrient goals and intermediate goals for the general population and the high-risk group. *Alcohol intake* should be limited. *Iodine prophylaxis* should be applied when necessary and *nutrient density* should be increased. Finally, a *body mass index (BMI)* of 20–25 is both an intermediate and an ultimate goal, although this value is not necessarily appropriate for the developing world, in which the average BMI may be 18.

diet and consider several aspects of health as well as the prevention of coronary heart disease. Worrying evidence shows that countries in eastern Europe are moving towards an unsatisfactory diet, similar to that of northern Europeans. The Mediterranean countries remain relatively fortunate, with a traditional pattern of foods that provides nutrient intakes very similar to the WHO goals, but, again, there is evidence of adverse change.

Governments should translate these nutrient goals into food goals and eventually into dietary guidelines relevant to their own dietary and cultural traditions, while taking into account the economic and other constraints on changes in the provision of food. A coherent food policy, taking prevention into account, involves joint action by ministries of health, agriculture, food, education, industry and economics if benefits to health are to be achieved without detriment to local food production. A combination of government action and education for individuals and for the community as a whole must be geared to the ability of the food and agricultural industries to make substantial adjustments in the provision of food. Provided each country develops a coherent and sustained nutrition policy, agricultural and food manufacturing practices can alter satisfactorily and remain profitable.

Health education in many forms will be required and will be more effective if it is based on an understanding of the links between diet and health. This book is therefore a prelude to other methods of informing policy-makers, health educators and the public about the lifestyles that are most conducive to a healthy adult life.

Introduction

In 1980 the WHO Regional Committee for Europe decided that specific regional targets should be formulated to support the European regional strategy for attaining health for all. In 1984 the same Committee adopted 38 regional targets to be reached by the year 2000.

Target 16 *(1)* is of specific relevance to people who are interested in nutrition, stating that:

> By 1995, in all Member States, there should be significant increases in positive health behaviour, such as balanced nutrition, nonsmoking, appropriate physical activity and good stress management.

A further specific objective is to assess the food and nutrition situation, to identify and promote policies and programmes that enhance health through appropriate nutrition.

In response to the need for action in this sphere, a Nutrition unit was created in the WHO Regional Office for Europe in September 1984. It has established a programme emphasizing the promotion of national policies on food and nutrition in Member States.

The remarkable increase in some chronic diseases over the last 35–40 years has increased the demand for government and international policies to encourage a preventive as well as therapeutic approach to these diseases and to limit their development in areas where their incidence is low.

This book highlights the rapidly growing evidence that poor diet and physical inactivity (as well as smoking, which is considered in other WHO publications) are important factors in the development of a variety of disorders that lead to substantial morbidity and mortality.

No group of medical experts or other official body would claim to know the precise mechanism whereby dietary factors lead to chronic diseases, but such a wealth of evidence now links diet to the pathophysiology of these conditions, that all European expert committees have called for public health policies to ensure that the people of Europe have access to and are able to choose a healthy diet.

There are two prerequisites for working out successful national food and nutrition strategies or policies. First, it is necessary to have a clear picture of a dietary pattern in a country and its associated public health

1

problems. Second, there must be sufficient agreement within the country on the nature of healthy nutrition, which is not necessarily a complicated problem since a consensus already seems to exist. This is made evident in the present publication, which sets out the current nutritional knowledge available in expert reports throughout the Region. The degree of unanimity in these reports should assure policy-makers that they can build their strategies on a sound basis.

The formulation of a nutrition strategy (a plan for handling the food supply that takes account of health) is a complex task that demands an understanding of all the principal factors invovled in the food chain. All Member States in the Region already have food policies in one form or another, which have an unintended effect on the health of the population. An explicit government nutrition policy requires a decision to develop a food policy with clear health objectives. The nutrition programme of the WHO Regional Office for Europe plans to analyse existing nutrition policies in a few selected European countries in the hope that this will stimulate other countries in the Region to develop their own nutrition strategies, which may in turn develop into government nutrition policies. A review of national strategies was begun in 1986.

Despite the diversity of dietary patterns in Europe, all population groups share common nutrient needs that must be met. It is important, therefore, to work out local dietary guidelines based on these common needs. Dietary guidelines must be based on a sound knowledge of local food patterns and take social and traditional values into account. A clear idea of what different groups of people actually consume is therefore essential.

Present knowledge of the diet and nutrient intake of different communities in Europe is based on a large number of individual studies made for a wide variety of reasons. There are no standardized studies on people's food consumption throughout Europe that can be used to produce compatible data on food or nutrient intake. For international comparisons of dietary patterns, data have therefore often been taken from the food balance sheets of the Food and Agriculture Organization of the United Nations (FAO). Although this macro-level analysis can serve a useful purpose in planning food and nutrition policies, it can give only a crude indication of actual dietary patterns, and the approach has several methodological weaknesses. Such analysis nevertheless reveals the patterns of food availability and their trends over time. To supplement this information, more precise dietary data have been used in this publication whenever possible.

This book was commissioned by WHO from a small group of medical nutritionists, and written in the course of 1985 and 1986. It was discussed with members of its potential audience on several occasions, to adjust its scope and presentation. The group drew on a wide range of sources to illustrate the nature of the problem to be tackled. The report produces a set of nutritional goals that European governments might use when considering how to develop their nutrition strategies. Dietary guidelines will, of course, vary from country to country.

Written by Professor W.P.T. James (in collaboration with Professor A. Ferro-Luzzi, Rome, Italy; Professor B. Isaksson, Gothenburg, Sweden; and

2

Professor W.B. Szostak, Warsaw, Poland), this book has benefited from the comments and advice of a wide range of professionals in public health, health education and nutrition.

The recommendations presented and views expressed reflect, whenever possible, those of government or other official reports; an attempt has been made to integrate the views of different national expert committees so that the final outcome represents as large a consensus as possible. Although the examples chosen to illustrate this consensus are inevitably based on the authors' experience, the views expressed are those of international and national bodies.

Aims and Scope

This book aims to provide a readable reference source for people formulating the objectives for nutrition policies in Europe. It also contains a brief résumé of the reasons that caused expert committees of WHO and of Member States to suggest that nutritional factors are important in the development of a number of the major diseases of significance to public health in Europe. Evidence on diet and disease is presented for mainly European countries; non-European literature is used when it helps to explain the link between nutrient intake and illness.

This book should not be seen as providing proof that diet is the principal factor in the etiology of these diseases. Nutrient goals are established by experts who collate evidence from clinical experience, pathological analyses, animal research, epidemiological surveys, metabolic studies and many controlled trials with hospital patients and population groups. If the evidence constituted proof of the precise role and importance of nutrition, there would have been little need for so many assessments. Some of the recommendations arising from these assessments are construed as controversial by individual investigators, but these experts are a small minority in Europe and North America. This report does not attempt to deal with all the concerns of these critics, nor does it set out the metabolic and biochemical evidence that underlies most of the recommendations.

This book does not deal with other aspects of preventive medicine, such as the need to persuade people not to smoke. Similarly, the maintenance of physical activity throughout adult life is recognized as an important factor in maintaining people's health and wellbeing, but this will not be discussed in any detail. The benefits of exercise to health have been set out elsewhere (2). The book concentrates on the epidemiological evidence of dietary patterns and disease and on the controlled dietary trials aimed at preventing disease in subsections of a population; eventually all proposals for dietary change must be tested in population groups or whole communities. It emphasizes the prevalence of nutrition-related disease in European countries and describes how European studies have helped to shed light on the role of diet. Comparisons of current dietary patterns are then related to the ultimate nutrient goals and a set of intermediate goals are developed based on national recommendations. These intermediate goals appear to be more appropriate for the northern European countries than for the rest of Europe,

3

where nutrient intakes are closer to those considered optimal for health. The pragmatic decisions of national committees in these northern countries are conditioned by the agricultural and economic problems that would ensue if rapid and major changes in dietary patterns occurred.

This publication does not review every nutrition topic that has concerned government policy-makers in the past, and it cannot be considered a textbook of nutrition. Other concerns that nutritionists usually deal with, such as food safety, are also excluded. The use of food additives and colouring agents is not mentioned, since the evidence that they constitute a public health problem is limited, unless salt and nitrite are considered as additives. Some additives, such as antioxidants and other food preservatives, have technological value but are not of direct relevance to nutrition. This conclusion does not deny the importance of the idiosyncratic responses of individuals to food additives and dietary components or the widespread concern among people in many countries about the use of food additives and colouring agents. Similarly, many vitamin and mineral deficiencies are of great general interest, but are considered much less important to public health in Europe than the diseases discussed here.

At present, the public and the health workers in many countries are very confused about nutrition and often continue to regard particular foods as having special and mysterious effects that promote health. Developing a more rational view will require a sustained educational programme. It is hoped that this book will contribute to a more balanced discussion of nutrition. A clear exposition of current nutritional knowledge is important and care should be taken not to claim too much. The recommendations summarized here will not, if implemented, provide a panacea for all ill health, but they could contribute substantially to reducing morbidity as well as rates of premature death in many European countries. A new concept of healthy nutrition is presented in accordance with target 16 of the WHO regional strategy for health for all.

This book can have many uses, some of which are illustrated in Fig. 1. Many short versions of it may be needed for different purposes, particularly if the concepts presented are to be set out for a wider audience.

Terminology: Balanced, Rational or simply a Healthy Diet?

Balanced diets have been a central theme of nutrition education programmes for many years. This concept of balance stems from recognition of the fact that an appropriate mixture of food items will provide at least the minimum requirements of protein, vitamins and minerals needed by the body; these requirements are less likely to be met if the diet contains only a few foods. By ensuring that several different foods are consumed, the idea is that one item rich in a particular nutrient will balance the lack of this nutrient in another food. The balanced diet is therefore a term that has arisen from a concern that a diet should prevent the development of deficiency diseases. The choice of a variety of foods also ensures that any toxic element in a single food will have a reduced impact.

Fig. 1. Uses and users of this book

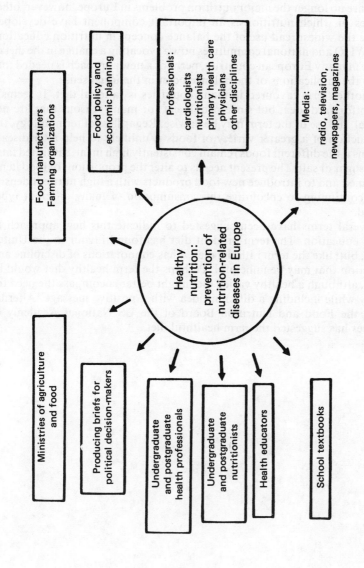

Food manufacturers
Farming organizations

Food policy and
economic planning

Professionals:
cardiologists
nutritionists
primary health care
physicians
other disciplines

Media:
radio, television,
newspapers, magazines

Ministries of agriculture
and food

Producing briefs for
political decision-makers

Undergraduate
and postgraduate
health professionals

Undergraduate
and postgraduate
nutritionists

Health educators

School textbooks

Healthy
nutrition:
prevention of
nutrition-related
diseases in Europe

It could well be argued that the reduction in the prevalence of deficiency diseases is in part a response to the concept of a balanced diet in nutrition education. Yet confusion remains, because many members of the public, and even people in nutrition education, view the balanced diet simply as a choice of foods needed to avoid vitamin, protein or mineral deficiencies. These are no longer the major nutrition problems in Europe, however; other diseases in which nutrition is an important component have developed despite the widespread use of the balance concept in nutrition education. With WHO and national committees now advocating a change in the diet of people in many European countries, perhaps a new approach is needed that avoids the implications of the balanced diet in the usual sense.

Another term favoured in many countries is rational diet. It seems a straightforward idea, but since people eat for many reasons that are not rational, the use of the term may be unwise. Regardless of terminology, the introduction of a greater variety of foods is unlikely to help alter disease patterns if the different foods remain consistently high in fat, saturated fatty acids, sugar or salt. The present need is to alter the proportions of food items consumed and to introduce new food products with a high nutrient density while continuing to encourage the consumption of many different types of food.

Several terms have been suggested to indicate this new approach to health education. The term prudent diet has found favour in the United States, but, like the term rational diet, it has connotations of discipline and restriction that may be unhelpful. Perhaps the term healthy diet would be useful, although a healthy varied diet might better encompass the need for variety while including a different idea with a positive message. Alternatively, the Food and Nutrition Board of the US National Academy of Sciences has suggested the term healthful diet.

Food patterns
in Europe

Traditions and Cultural Variety

Travellers have recognized for centuries the extraordinary diversity of food patterns across the continent of Europe. The traditional cuisines of different countries are intrinsic features of their cultures and have been developed and refined over many generations. The need for maximum use of local produce and for variety in the diet has frequently stimulated the development of skills for producing different dishes. The customs of preserving and processing food, such as those used in fermenting milk, making cheese, and cooking and presenting food, are often so localized that a journey through a single country can reveal a myriad of dishes, some of which are as unfamiliar to the inhabitants of other regions of the country as they are to foreigners. Traditional dishes also show a marked seasonal pattern in keeping with the availability of cereals, fruit, vegetables and animal products. To cope with winter, a variety of strategies has been developed in different localities to maintain the quality of foods that are dried, salted or preserved by other means. Folklore, slowly evolved, often dominates traditional methods of food preservation and preparation, emphasizing specific methods so as to maintain not only the palatability of the food but also its safety and health-promoting properties.

Recognizing that the type as well as the quantity of food is important for health has been an important feature of most cultures. The supposed link between food and health formed the basis of much medical practice and thinking before the advent of scientific medicine and drug therapy. The discovery of vitamins and of the effects of mineral deficiencies in the early part of this century confirmed the widely held belief that an adequate variety of foods was conducive to the growth of healthy children and the welfare of adults. The early research on the biochemical role of vitamins and minerals was rapidly transferred into medical practice and into the making of government food policies.

So successful was the application of hygienic principles in public health that it soon became evident that bacteriological and nutritional problems in the community could be solved by the avoidance of bacteriologically contaminated food and the provision of a diet adequate in energy, protein, vitamins and minerals. Nutritional surveillance, including monitoring the growth of children and the weight and height of adults, became a recognized tool for assessing public health and the impact of changes in national food supply. These anthropometric measures were a more precise indicator of nutritional adequacy than statistics on the cause of death in children and adults. By the late 1930s, many national programmes on nutrition and health surveillance included the collection of statistics on causes of death, on food patterns of different groups within society, and on the growth of children and the weight and height of adults.

Following the Second World War, Europe underwent a period of some 5–10 years during which food supplies were barely sufficient while major economic recovery and industrial reconstruction took place. Conditions steadily improved, and the variety and quality of food supplies ensured that nutritional deficiencies were minimized. Thereafter, for about a quarter of a century, the emphasis was on maintaining this progress. As the numbers of people diagnosed with overt vitamin and most mineral deficiencies (except iron deficiency) fell, emphasis on nutritional surveillance declined. These classic techniques for monitoring nutritional status were, however, taken up in the developing world, where they are still given prime importance in determining the distribution and nature of medical and nutritional support.

Some physicians in Europe have reintroduced the traditional practice of prescribing diets for the treatment of many diseases, but the therapy now reflects the development of a scientific approach. The re-emergence of nutritional counselling has been slow because, in the last 40 years, the power of antibiotics and other drugs has appeared sufficient for disease management and has therefore dominated medical practice. Public health programmes therefore still centre mainly on the provision of a good immunization programme for children, on the maintenance of safe water and food supplies, free from toxins and bacterial contamination, and on the provision of suitable facilities for the care of the rapidly expanding elderly population.

Dietary Surveillance in Europe

In view of the recognized variety of diet even within one country, any attempt at a synthesis of the wealth of information on European diets might seem foolish. Certainly, doing justice to the complexity of culinary practices is impossible, since this would involve a country-by-country analysis with regional or even district monitoring of food consumption throughout the year. It would be equally impossible to monitor individual food consumption for a sufficient time to obtain a comprehensive view of the intake of dietary components of biological significance throughout the year, although this would be the perfect answer. On the other hand, a simple collation of food types would be incomplete because anomalies in nutrition would arise from differences in methods of preparing and cooking food.

Table 2 illustrates the major sources of dietary information used in nutritional surveillance. The crude statistics based on food production in a country are modified to take account of food imports and exports and

8

Table 2. Major sources of dietary information

Parts of the food chain surveyed	Type of data published	Scope and limitations of survey data
National food supply	Food balance data collected by agriculture ministries, collated by FAO	Allows for home production, imports and exports, changing food stocks
Market distribution	Industrial data	Limited to specific sectors
Household budget	Economic statistics	Limited to financial outlay of whole households on food; costs do not relate to nutritional value of purchases
Household consumption	Household food survey	Often fails to allow for food eaten elsewhere; food waste assumed
Individual nutrition	Individual food and nutrient intake	Numerous methods available of varying reliability

are collected annually by most ministries of agriculture for collation, standardization and presentation as food balance sheets on a common basis by the Food and Agriculture Organization of the United Nations (FAO). These figures encompass regional and seasonal variations; they take account of waste during the marketing and distribution of food but not that in home preparation and consumption. They therefore substantially overestimate total food intake.

Other statistical information comes from market, household budget and household food surveys. Each of these is a more refined indicator of nutrient intake and dietary patterns, but none can compete with the quality of data collected on the food consumption of individuals. Nevertheless, the overall range of national dietary patterns can be illustrated by collating all the sources of food, country by country, and expressing this in terms of the population. These data are given in the FAO food balance sheets.

European Food Supplies

Recent statistics from FAO reveal remarkable differences in food supply in different countries (3). These can be expressed simply by recalculating the data to show the proportion of total food energy derived from different food sources. Fig. 2 shows the proportion of energy derived from vegetable and

Fig. 2. Total energy available per capita per day from vegetable and animal products, and from alcohol in European countries, 1979–1981

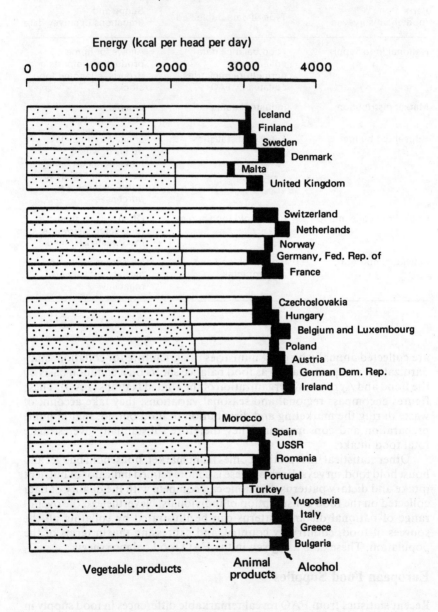

Energy (kcal per head per day)

Note. These data may be subject to errors and approximations.

Source: Food balance sheets, 1979–81 average (3).

10

animal products and alcohol by each country. A few countries in the WHO European Region do not have data that can be expressed in this way, but there is sufficient coverage to reveal geographical differences. The northern countries and the United Kingdom have the lowest provision of vegetable products, this perhaps reflecting the climatic limitations on growing cereals, roots, fruit and vegetables. In contrast, the Mediterranean countries and those in the eastern parts of Europe have predominantly vegetable sources of energy, with animal products making a smaller contribution.

A more detailed picture of this phenomenon can be seen in Fig. 3, which shows the range of fruit and vegetable consumption in different countries,

Fig. 3. Energy derived from fruit and vegetables
in European countries, 1979–1981

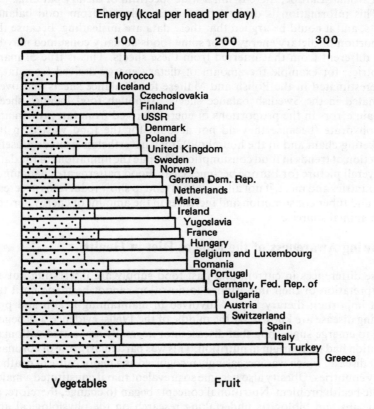

Note. These data may be subject to errors and approximations.

Source: Food balance sheets, 1979–81 average (3).

11

expressed for simplicity in terms of the energy provided by each category *(3)*. Roots and tubers have been arbitrarily excluded from the vegetable category. There are clearly remarkable differences in the availability of fruit and vegetables, with Greece having more than three times as much as is available in Morocco. The differences are reflected in both fruit and vegetable consumption, although countries vary widely in the dominance of one source rather than another. Nevertheless, as expected, the fruits make a greater contribution of energy than the vegetables.

When earlier food balance sheets are consulted, it becomes clear that food intake has changed strikingly in many countries over the last 20 years. This is illustrated in Fig. 4 by the changes in intake of selected foods in Denmark, Hungary, Portugal and Switzerland (one country from each of the arbitrary groupings shown in Fig. 2). In general, the production of cereals, roots and tubers for human consumption has declined while that of animal products such as meat has steadily risen. Fruit and vegetables are becoming more readily available but, despite an increase in the movement of food around Europe, there is still a wide spectrum of dietary patterns.

This information is derived from data collected from food balance sheets, and it could be argued that these data are misleading, because the proportion of dietary energy from some foods actually consumed may be very different from that inferred from these sheets. This is true of many countries; for example the amount of dietary energy derived from fat is underestimated in the Polish and Maltese food balance sheets and overestimated in the Swedish balance sheets. Although food balance sheets contain errors in the proportions of energy derived from fat, protein and carbohydrate (because they do not account for the food wasted in the marketing chain and in the household), they nevertheless provide a useful reflection of trends in food consumption. Despite the limitations of the data, an overall picture for Europe becomes clear. Food patterns are changing in all countries and most, if not all, countries tend to show reductions in cereal, root and tuber consumption and increases in the amount of energy derived from animal sources.

Growing Awareness of the Role of Diet in Health

These differences in current and past food supply are interesting but an interpretation of their importance to nutrition cannot be made until the most important dietary factors involved in maintaining health and preventing disease are known. By the middle of the 1960s, evidence was beginning to emerge suggesting that diseases not normally associated with malnutrition had their origin in nutrition. This was particularly true of coronary heart disease, which was increasingly recognized as a major cause of death in many countries. Obesity also became so prevalent that it constituted a major public health problem. Nutritional concepts began to change, therefore, as physicians and biologists undertaking research on the physiological and biochemical basis of chronic degenerative diseases slowly realized that nutrient intakes might be linked to a number of risk factors and to the development of such diverse conditions as coronary heart disease, gallstones

12

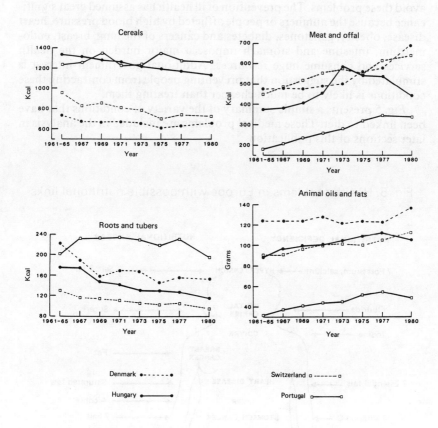

Fig. 4. Changes in intake of selected foods in Denmark, Hungary, Portugal and Switzerland (per capita per day)

Source: FAO food balance sheets (1961–1980).

and cancer of the colon. Nutritional excesses, as well as deficiencies of, for example, iodine and iron, were now considered worthy of study. In addition, renewed interest arose in the concept of fibre deficiency, stimulated by physicians returning from Africa and Asia where dietary patterns were so different, and where many of the major European diseases were rarely seen except in a small group of affluent people with refined European diets.

In the last 20 years, there has been an upsurge in nutritional research and the findings, though incomplete, are sufficiently convincing for many government committees to call for changes in national diets. Evidence of the importance of nutritional factors varies widely, and rarely is it sufficient to satisfy rigorous clinical examination. Nevertheless, the medical problems involved are of such importance to public health that expert committees of governments and such interested bodies as WHO have recommended substantial changes in the diet of the European population in an attempt to avoid these problems. The prevention of ill health has assumed great significance because the numbers of people afflicted by high blood pressure, heart disease, obesity, gallstones, diabetes and cancers of the lung, breast, endometrium, intestine and stomach impose a major burden on the health services and consume huge resources. Additional government interest is stimulated by the suggestion that preventing people from contracting these conditions is likely to be much cheaper than treating them.

Fig. 5 presents a simple summary of the variety of conditions that have been linked to diet. These medical problems are included in the analysis in later sections of this publication.

Fig. 5. Health problems in Europe with possible nutritional links

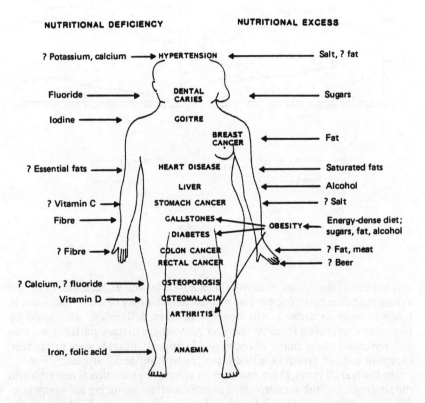

Note. Individual susceptibility to the prevailing diet is important in both nutritional deficiency and excess. The nutritional components have only been tentatively linked to many of the conditions shown.

The nature of
the public health problem

No policy on the prevention of a disease can be developed without a realistic assessment of its prevalence and its impact on morbidity and mortality, and an estimate of the possible outcome of implementing defined preventive measures. Unfortunately, there are few standardized data on the morbidity of the European population, which in 1980 was estimated at 815 million (4). Therefore, reliance here is placed initially on mortality data recently collated by Brzeziński for the WHO Regional Office for Europe.[a] A limited selection of these data has been made simply to illustrate the principal problems to be tackled.

Diseases of infancy and childhood are no longer the scourge of Europe: only 3% of all deaths occur in children below the age of 15 years (who make up one quarter of the population). Some 24% of deaths occur in men and women below the age of 65 years; these deaths can readily be considered premature. If their causes are known, preventive measures can be identified and implemented.

It is traditionally considered that preventive measures in the elderly (people aged over 65 years) may be misplaced; some national committees (5) recommend less attention to this age group in preventive medicine. Yet recently a WHO working group[b] concluded that attempts should be made to prevent cardiovascular disease by nutritional means in the elderly as well as in the younger age groups, the aim being to maintain good health into later life, to reduce disability and thereby to decrease the burden on society.

Fig. 6 and 7 demonstrate that in middle-aged and elderly men and women, there are up to twofold differences in the rate of premature death in different European countries. The grouping of data has also been made to show that the countries with a high death rate in the middle-aged also have high death rates in the elderly; these data apply to people up to 84 years old. This explains in part the distinct variations in the number of very old people

---

[a] **Brzeziński, Z.J.** *Regional targets in support of the regional strategy for health for all: epidemiological background.* Copenhagen, WHO Regional Office for Europe, 1984 (unpublished document EUR/RC34/Conf.Doc./5).

[b] *Nutrition in the elderly.* Copenhagen, WHO Regional Office for Europe, 1987 (unpublished document IRP/HEE 114.2.5).

Fig. 6. Standardized mortality rates per 100 000 population, males, 1975–1979, all causes

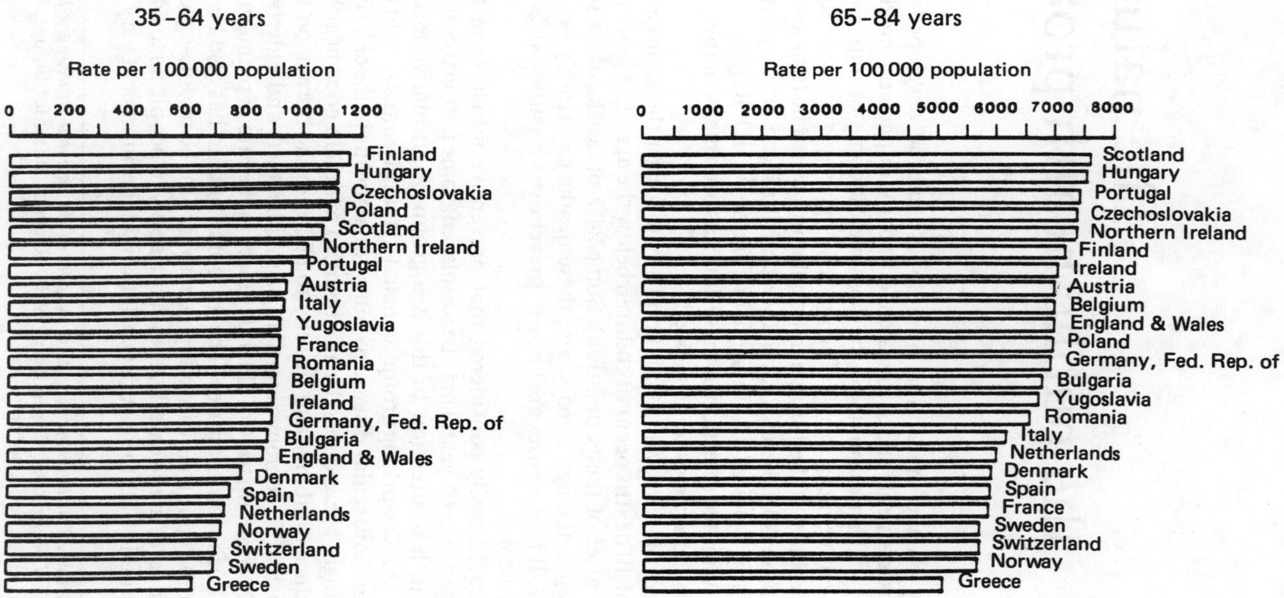
35–64 years
Rate per 100 000 population
0
200
400
600
800
1000
1200
Finland
Hungary
Czechoslovakia
Poland
Scotland
Northern Ireland
Portugal
Austria
Italy
Yugoslavia
France
Romania
Belgium
Ireland
Germany, Fed. Rep. of
Bulgaria
England & Wales
Denmark
Spain
Netherlands
Norway
Switzerland
Sweden
Greece
65–84 years
Rate per 100 000 population
0
1000
2000
3000
4000
5000
6000
7000
8000
Scotland
Hungary
Portugal
Czechoslovakia
Northern Ireland
Finland
Ireland
Austria
Belgium
England & Wales
Poland
Germany, Fed. Rep. of
Bulgaria
Yugoslavia
Romania
Italy
Netherlands
Denmark
Spain
France
Sweden
Switzerland
Norway
Greece

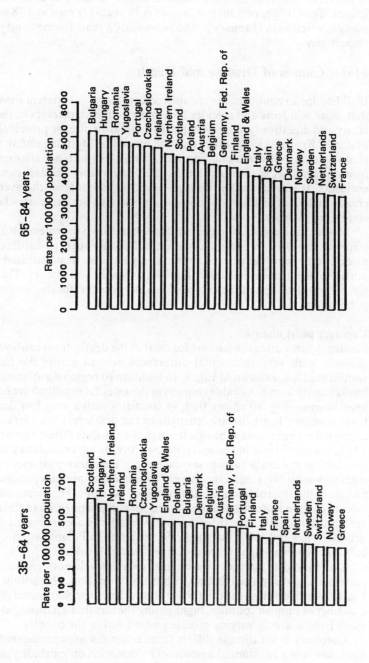

Fig. 7. Standardized mortality rates per 100 000 population, females, 1975–1979, all causes

65–84 years

Rate per 100 000 population

Bulgaria
Hungary
Romania
Yugoslavia
Portugal
Czechoslovakia
Ireland
Northern Ireland
Scotland
Poland
Austria
Belgium
Germany, Fed. Rep. of
Finland
England & Wales
Italy
Spain
Greece
Denmark
Norway
Sweden
Netherlands
Switzerland
France

35–64 years

Rate per 100 000 population

Scotland
Hungary
Northern Ireland
Ireland
Romania
Czechoslovakia
Yugoslavia
England & Wales
Poland
Bulgaria
Denmark
Belgium
Austria
Germany, Fed. Rep. of
Portugal
Finland
Italy
France
Spain
Netherlands
Sweden
Switzerland
Norway
Greece

17

in different countries and the variable life expectancy in different populations. Thus, life expectancy in Greece is 73 years for men and 78 years for women, whereas in Hungary it is 66 years and 73 years for men and women, respectively.

Major Causes of Disease and Death

If all European countries are considered together it is apparent from Fig. 8 that, once accidents and suicides have been excluded, diseases of the circulatory and digestive systems, along with neoplasms, are the principal causes of death. Brzeziński suggested that the impact of lifestyle-related diseases could be assessed by recalculating the data on life expectancy after removing from the analysis cardiovascular diseases, respiratory disease, cancer and accidents. If cardiovascular diseases alone are eliminated, the average increase in life expectancy in Europe amounts to seven years; the other conditions have less impact.

Medical and epidemiological evidence has shown the role of nutrition in some of the most prevalent diseases in Europe, such as cardiovascular diseases and some cancers. Scientific study has also demonstrated the importance of nutrition in such conditions as goitre and obesity. These considerations determined the choice of health problems for discussion in this publication.

Coronary heart disease
Coronary heart disease accounts for most of the deaths from cardiovascular diseases, with very substantial differences evident across the European continent. This is shown in Fig. 9. In addition to regional variations, there have recently been noticeable changes in the rate of mortality from coronary heart disease. Fig. 10 shows that, in countries with a very low death rate from coronary heart disease, changes in the death rate are marked when expressed on a percentage basis, although the absolute differences are small. The fall in death rates in Finland is noteworthy, however, and the increase of over 50% in the death rates in several eastern European countries contrasts markedly with the trend elsewhere. These changes are independent of revisions in the International Classification of Diseases. The increasing death rates in eastern Europe have been noted for some time (6,7). In Poland, the age-adjusted death rate from coronary heart disease increased by 65% between 1969 and 1977, but the 1979 death rate in Poland was only about half that observed eight years earlier in Czechoslovakia.

The marked differences from country to country do not signify a uniform pattern of coronary heart disease within any one nation. This is illustrated in Fig. 11, which displays the range of mortality from coronary heart disease in a number of Finnish counties, highlighting the fact that a national average is made from a widely varying disease pattern within the country.

Coronary heart disease differs from other diseases considered in this book, because a substantial amount of information on morbidity as well as mortality is now available through the myocardial infarction community registers that form part of the WHO project on the multinational monitoring

18

Fig. 8. Causes of loss of potential life up to 65 years
(latest available data, around 1980)

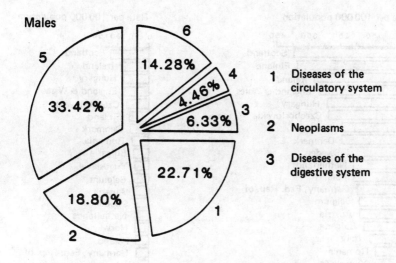

Males

6 14.28%

5 33.42%

4 4.46%

3 6.33%

22.71% 1

18.80%

2

1 Diseases of the circulatory system

2 Neoplasms

3 Diseases of the digestive system

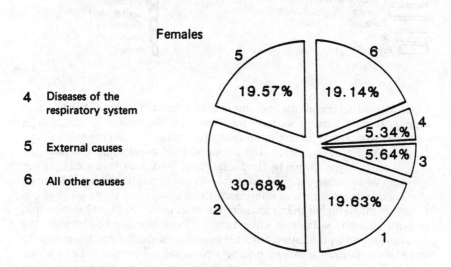

Females

5 19.57%

6 19.14%

4 5.34%

3 5.64%

30.68%

19.63%

2

1

4 Diseases of the respiratory system

5 External causes

6 All other causes

19

Fig. 9. Ischaemic heart disease: standardized mortality rates
per 100 000 population, 1980

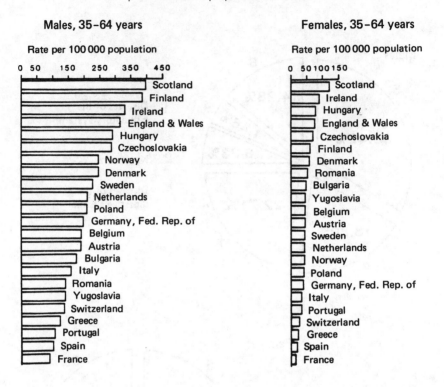

Males, 35–64 years

Rate per 100 000 population

Females, 35–64 years

Rate per 100 000 population

of trends and determinants in cardiovascular disease (MONICA) *(9)*. These employ standardized procedures for identifying the annual incidence rates of acute myocardial infarction in many communities, ranging from Perth, Scotland to Tel Aviv, Israel. The importance of monitoring morbidity as well as mortality is shown by the finding that there are over twice as many episodes of acute myocardial infarction in the community as deaths from this condition. Myocardial infarction is not always lethal; its incidence is therefore much higher than mortality statistics indicate. Fig. 12 shows that, in both men and women in cities ranging from Warsaw to Helsinki, the relationship on a population basis between the morbidity and the mortality from this condition seems surprisingly consistent. The medical and social problems of coronary heart disease therefore include the substantial effects of illness and residual disability as well as those of premature mortality.

A consistent feature of the statistical analysis of morbidity and mortality is that, throughout Europe, the death rates from coronary heart disease in women have declined. The pattern of heart disease in men differs considerably from that in women and mortality from this cause is substantially higher in men in every European country (see Fig. 9).

20

Fig. 10. Average percentage change in mortality
from coronary heart disease
for males aged 40–69 years, 1968–1977

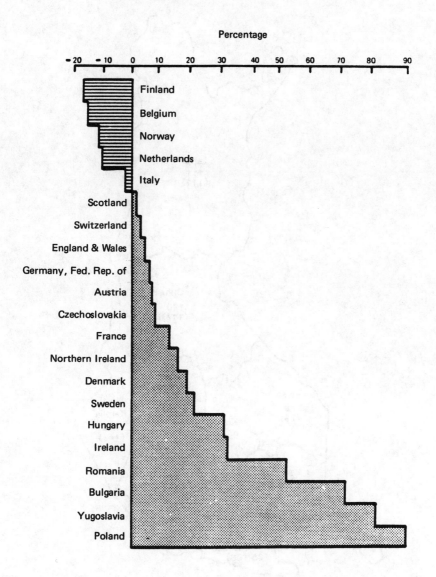

Note. Percentages are based on the slopes of linear regressions fitted to mortality trends in the six quinquennial age groups.

Source: Pisa & Uemura *(7).*

Fig. 11. Age-standardized mortality from coronary heart disease
for males aged 35–64 years
in different counties of Finland, 1979–1981

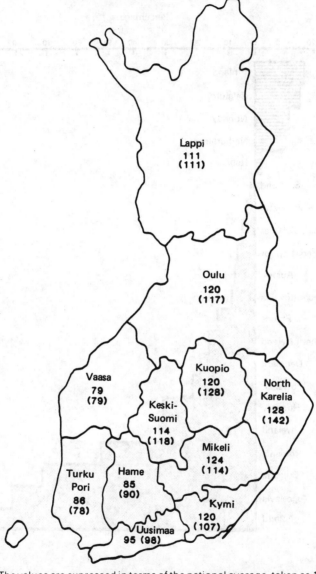

Note. The values are expressed in terms of the national average, taken as 100. Values in brackets are those observed 10 years earlier. Data are recalculated and are three-year average death rates. The national death rate from coronary heart disease was 504 in 1969–1971 and 409 in 1979–1981.

Source: Pyorala et al. *(8).*

22

Fig. 12. Correlation between the attack rate of
acute myocardial infarction computed from the registers
and the death rate from category 410 of the ICD (Eighth revision),
as given in the national vital statistics: 55–64 years

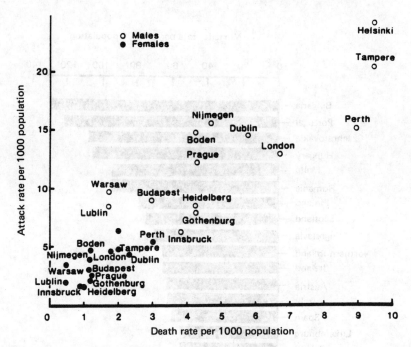

Source: Lamm *(10).*

Cerebrovascular disease

Brzeziński[a] noted that cerebrovascular disease is the second most important cause of cardiovascular mortality. Mortality from both coronary heart and cerebrovascular disease differs widely between European countries, as do the patterns of disease. Many of the countries with a high death rate from stroke have a relatively low death rate from heart disease. The differences in the incidence of coronary heart disease and that of stroke in both men and women are evident even in young and middle-aged adults, aged 35–64 years. The incidence of stroke is changing in Europe, resulting in a rising death rate in eastern European countries and a decline in death rates in northern Europe (Fig. 13 and 14).

[a] **Brzeziński, Z.J.** *Regional targets in support of the regional strategy for health for all: epidemiological background.* Copenhagen, WHO Regional Office for Europe, 1984 (unpublished document EUR/RC34/Conf.Doc./5).

Fig. 13. Cerebrovascular disease: standardized mortality rates
per 100 000 population,
males, 35–64 years, 1975–1979

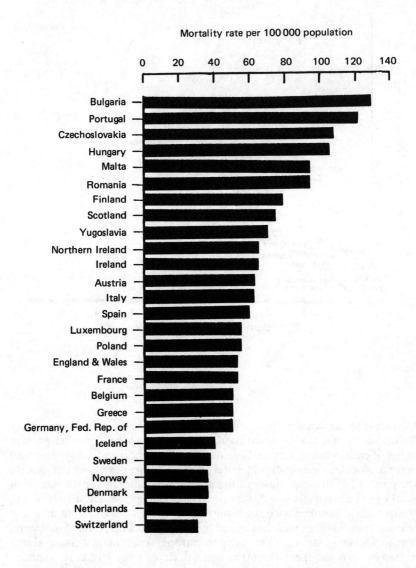

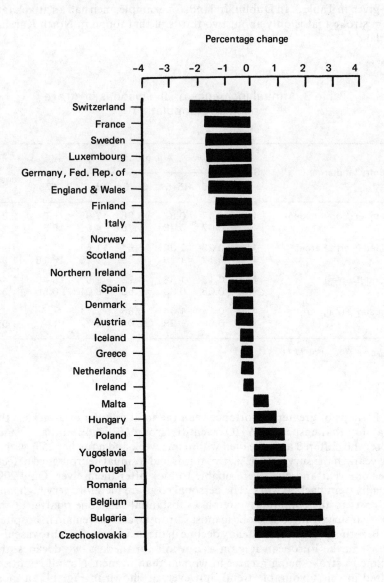

Fig. 14. Cerebrovascular disease: annual percentage change
in standardized mortality rates per 100 000 population,
males, 35–64 years from 1955–1959 to 1975–1979

A community-based register has been used for assessing cerebrovascular morbidity in 17 centres *(11)*. In the seven European centres, the annual rate for stroke for all age groups ranged from 1.5 to 2.5 per 1000 population; incidence increased with age. Some of the differences shown by this study are given in Table 3. In Dublin, Ireland, for example, men had an attack rate from stroke that is only about two thirds of that found in North Karelia, Finland.

Table 3. Annual incidence of all episodes of stroke
per 1000 population

Country (and area)	Sex	Age group (years)					All ages
		<45	45–54	55–64	65–74	≧75	
Denmark (Copenhagen)	M	0.07	0.82	3.88	7.65	15.04	2.37
	F	0.07	0.48	1.76	4.65	15.35	2.70
Finland (North Karelia)	M	0.22	2.82	5.61	11.51	18.16	1.96
	F	0.17	1.29	3.89	9.35	18.18	1.98
Ireland (Dublin)	M	0.13	1.38	4.73	9.50	18.40	1.44
	F	0.06	0.83	2.60	8.01	20.56	1.58
Yugoslavia (Zagreb)	M	0.14	1.64	4.66	7.71	N/A	2.23
	F	0.09	1.28	2.05	4.72	N/A	1.90

Source: Aho et al. *(11)*.

Perhaps of greater importance than the total number of attacks is the disability that ensues. A WHO scientific group *(12)* showed that 23% of those who suffered a stroke died within one week and a further 25% within one year. Of the surviving 52%, two thirds had residual neurological defects after one year and 40% were unable to look after themselves. Only 20% actually went back to work. The personal costs are therefore very high, and the costs to the community are also substantial since one quarter of the one-year survivors from stroke in most European centres remain in hospital.

Brzeziński has noted a steady decline in the incidence of cerebrovascular disease in the European Region as a whole for the last two decades, the decline in stroke being greater in women than in men. Not all countries shared in this favourable trend, however, as shown in Fig. 14. In most countries, the decline of stroke in women has meant that a greater difference in its incidence according to gender is becoming apparent.

The changing incidence of stroke, and the substantial differences in the rates of stroke among and within countries suggest that, as with heart disease, environmental factors play a substantial part in determining the changing rate of cerebrovascular disease. Possible environmental factors are considered later in this publication.

Diabetes

WHO recently analysed the problem of diabetes mellitus on a worldwide basis *(13)*. The definition of diabetes is important because the numbers of people classified as having diabetes vary with the criteria used; Table 4 summarizes the criteria, using a standard protocol, agreed on by a WHO study group. In addition, a large number of people have impaired glucose tolerance, a glycaemic response to a standard glucose challenge that falls between the responses of normal and diabetic individuals. The term impaired glucose tolerance replaces others such as borderline diabetes, pre-diabetes and chemical diabetes.

Major geographical and ethnic differences exist in the prevalence of insulin-dependent diabetes mellitus (Tables 5 and 6) and non-insulin-dependent diabetes mellitus. There is clearly a peak age for the clinical presentation of insulin-dependent diabetes, and for some unexplained reason it appears to be the age of 10–13 years with, in Europe, a clear relationship between the possession of some genes in a major histocompatibility group and the risk of diabetes. Thus, the possession of HLA-DR3 and/or HLA-DR4 alleles of the major histocompatibility complex on chromosome 6 is a marker of genetic susceptibility to insulin-dependent diabetes mellitus. The factors that precipitate diabetes in these genetically susceptible individuals remain somewhat uncertain, but viral infections are increasingly thought to play a leading role.

No specific genetic marker has been found for non-insulin-dependent diabetes but, because there are high rates of concordance in monozygotic twins, some genetic basis is presumably involved. In Europe, however, the prevalence of non-insulin-dependent diabetes mellitus (accounting for 80% of diabetics in the population) begins to rise at about the age of 40 years. Fig. 15 shows the grouping of prevalence rates in Europe. The classification was developed to take account of the marked variations in diabetes throughout the world. It is evident that diabetes mellitus in the European Region has a fairly consistent prevalence rate of 2–5%. The exceptions are Malta and Sweden, with prevalence rates in adults of 5–10%, and Israel, with a rate of 10–20%. These rates are well in excess of those found in Africa; in general, Caucasians are considered to have the highest rates.

Cancer

Of all cancer deaths in Europe, those in men most often result from cancer of the bronchus and lung (33%). Cancer of the lip, oral cavity, pharynx, larynx and oesophagus makes up 12% of the total, followed by cancer of the stomach (11%); intestine, colon and rectum (8%); and lymphatic and haemopoetic tissue (6%). Other cancers (of the brain, skin or bladder) comprise the remaining 30% of cancer deaths in men. In women, the pattern is a little different, with cancer of the breast being the dominant single cancer (24%), followed by cancer of the intestine, colon and rectum (10%); bronchus and

27

Table 4. Diagnostic values for the oral glucose tolerance test

| | Glucose concentration, mmol/litre (mg/dl) | | | | |
| | Whole blood | | Plasma | | |
	Venous	Capillary	Venous	Capillary
Diabetes mellitus				
Fasting value[a]	≧ 6.7 (≧ 120)	≧ 6.7 (≧ 120)	≧ 7.8 (≧ 140)	≧ 7.8 (≧ 140)
Two hours after glucose load[a]	≧ 10.0 (≧ 180)	≧ 11.1 (≧ 200)	≧ 11.1 (≧ 200)	≧ 12.2 (≧ 200)
Impaired glucose tolerance				
Fasting value[a]	< 6.7 (< 120)	< 6.7 (< 120)	< 7.8 (< 140)	< 7.8 (< 140)
Two hours after glucose load[a]	6.7–10.0 (120–180)	7.8–11.1 (140–200)	7.8–11.1 (140–200)	8.9–12.2 (160–220)

[a] For epidemiological or population screening purposes, the two-hour value after 75 g oral glucose may be used alone or with the fasting value. The fasting value alone is considered less reliable, since true fasting cannot be assured and spurious diagnosis of diabetes may more readily occur.

Source: WHO Technical Report Series, No. 727, p. 11 *(13)*.

Table 5. Prevalence of insulin-dependent diabetes in certain populations, 1970–1980

Location	Age group studied (years)	Method of ascertainment	Prevalence (per 1000 population)
China	10–19	Survey	0.09
Cuba	0–15	National registry	0.14
France	0–19	Central registry	0.32
Japan	7–15	School records	0.07
Scandinavian countries	0–14	National registry of hospital records	0.83–2.23
United Kingdom	0–26	National survey of health and development	3.40
United States	5–17	School records	1.93

Source: WHO Technical Report Series, No. 727, p. 103 (13).

Table 6. Incidence of insulin-dependent diabetes
in certain populations, 1970–1980

Location	Period of study	Age group studied (years)	Incidence (per 100 000 person-years at risk)
Canada (Toronto)	1976–1980	0–18	9
Finland	1970–1979	0–19	27
Israel: Ashkenazim	1975–1980	0–20	6.3
Non-Ashkenazim	1975–1980	0–20	2.6
Netherlands	1978–1980	0–19	11
Sweden (north)	1973–1977	0–14	38
United Kingdom (Scotland)	1968–1976	0–18	14
United States (Rhode Island)	1979–1980	0–29	14

Source: WHO Technical Report Series, No. 727, p. 103 (13).

lung (8%); stomach (7%); cervix uteri (6%); and lymphatic and haemopoetic tissue (6%). Other cancers account for the remaining 39%.

Lung cancer
Smoking is by far the most important factor promoting the development of lung cancer. Extensive studies around the world have established the evidence for this environmental cause of death, disease and disability. Numerous national and international documents have summarized this research. No further comment will therefore be made although there has been a suggestion that dietary factors may modify the effects of smoking; perhaps a higher carotene intake has a protective effect (14).

Breast cancer
The remarkable differences in the rates of mortality from breast cancer in different parts of Europe is shown in Fig. 16. Breast cancer rates in Britain and Ireland are more than twice those found in eastern Europe. Fig. 17 shows the annual percentage changes in standard mortality rates from 1955 to 1979. Death rates are still increasing in the United Kingdom, but on a percentage basis the increases are much greater in eastern Europe and the Mediterranean countries. Once more, environmental factors must clearly be very important.

Cancer of the oesophagus
The remarkable variation in death rates for cancer of the oesophagus found in European countries indicates a strong likelihood of an environmental

30

Fig. 15. Prevalence of diabetes mellitus in the WHO European Region

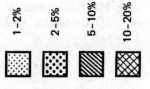

1–2%　2–5%　5–10%　10–20%

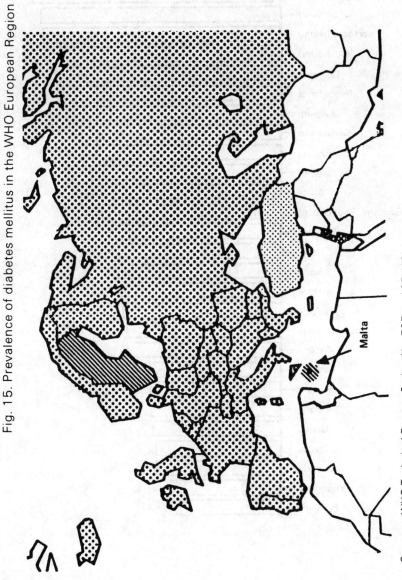

Malta

Source: WHO Technical Reports Series. No. 727. p. 105 *(13)*.

Fig. 16. Breast cancer: standardized mortality rates
per 100 000 population,
females, 30–64 years, 1975–1979

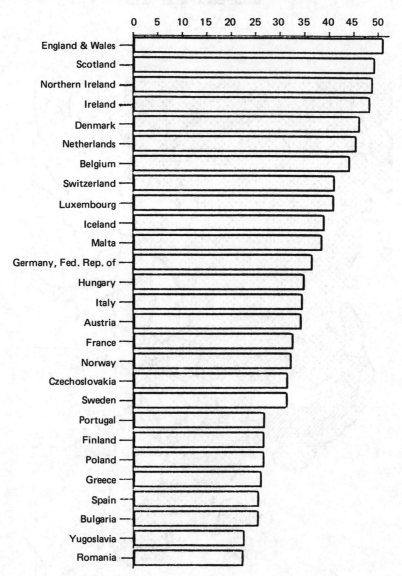

Mortality rate per 100 000 population

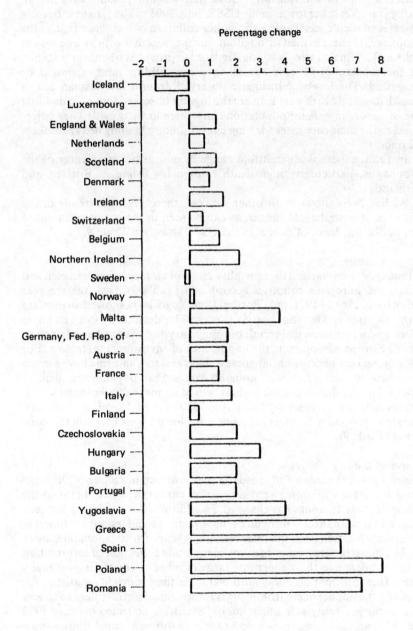

Fig. 17. Breast cancer: annual percentage changes
in standardized mortality rates per 100 000 population,
females, 30-64 years, from 1955-1959 to 1975-1979

Percentage change

basis for the differences; the extensive studies conducted in western and eastern Europe suggest several causes, rather than one specific cause, for this condition. For example, Cook-Mozaffari (15) noted an incidence rate in Gurjev, a town in Kazakhstan, USSR, that was comparable with that in nearby Iran. Yet other towns in the USSR, only 800 km away, have extremely low rates of incidence. Table 7 shows her collation of incidence figures for oesophageal cancer in men throughout Europe, together with an assessment of the male/female ratio. National figures are provided whenever possible, but the substantial differences among areas within countries should be recognized. The levels of incidence observed around the Caspian Sea in Kazakhstan and north-east Iran are the highest observed for any individual type of cancer in general populations anywhere in the world. They correspond to the incidence rates for lung cancer among lifelong heavy smokers in London.

In France there is an eightfold range in mortality from cancer of the oesophagus, particularly high death rates being found in Brittany and Normandy.

As has been shown with other cancers, there are time trends in the incidence of oesophageal cancer, as can be seen in the recent collation of data on the incidence of cancer in the USSR shown in Table 8.

Stomach cancer
Tulinius (17) summarized the mortality rates for stomach cancer in men and ranked the European countries accordingly (Table 9). Over the ten-year period from 1961 to 1971, only Portugal and Yugoslavia showed an increase in the mortality rate from gastric cancer. The declining rates elsewhere reflect an almost universal trend, but they vary widely. Studies performed outside Europe demonstrate the importance of environmental factors. For example, second-generation Japanese immigrants to California have a much lower rate of mortality from stomach cancer than Japanese resident in Japan (Fig. 18). Japan has the highest rate of stomach cancer in the world, but this decreased slightly (by 11%) from 1960 to 1970. In Iceland, however, the rate of mortality from gastric cancer declined by 46% during the same period (Table 9).

Cancer of the large bowel
Epidemiological analyses of trends in the incidence of cancer of the large bowel are not as straightforward as those for cancers of other organs, as the coding of these tumours has changed. In addition, distinguishing between colon and rectal cancer is difficult because rectosigmoid lesions are found in both types. Nevertheless, the International Agency for Research on Cancer (IARC) has strongly encouraged the meticulous collection of information on the incidence of this cancer in a large number of countries over many years. This information is far more valuable than mortality statistics for assessing the impact of environmental factors, since the treatment of cancer reduces the mortality rate substantially. Statistics, collected between 1973 and 1977, on the incidence of colon cancer in different communities show that it differs strikingly among countries and between urban and rural

34

Table 7. Incidence of cancer of the oesophagus per 100 000 population aged 35–64 years in Europe, as reported in studies made between 1966 and 1976

Country or area	Males	Male/female ratio
Eastern Europe		
Bulgaria	2.5[a,b]	2.0
Czechoslovakia	3.3[a]	5.4
German Democratic Republic	3.8	5.4
Hungary (Vas)	2.7	9.0[c]
Poland (Warsaw)	9.7	4.0
Romania (Banat)	2.3	7.7
Northern Europe		
Denmark	3.7	4.1
Finland	8.1	1.8
Iceland	3.4	1.8
Norway (urban)	4.6	7.7
Sweden	3.5	3.2
Southern Europe		
Italy	6.5[a]	5.7
Malta	3.4	8.5[c]
Portugal	11.5[a]	3.7
Spain (Zaragoza)	6.5	9.2
Yugoslavia (Slovenia)	9.6	16.0
Western Europe		
Austria	4.9[a]	6.5
Belgium	6.2[a]	4.9
France (Brittany and Normandy)	40.8[a,b]	25.0
Germany, Federal Republic of (Hamburg)	3.7	3.4
Netherlands (three provinces)	2.5	3.2
Switzerland (Geneva)	11.2	11.5
United Kingdom (average of six registers)	5.6	1.4
Southern USSR		
Georgia (urban)	7.9	5.1
Kazakhstan (Gurjev)	547.2	1.6
Western USSR (urban)		
Byelorussia	9.3[a,b]	3.6
Estonia	15.0[a,b]	7.2
Lithuania	5.2[a,b]	2.4
RSFSR	24.1[a,b]	9.8
Ukraine	10.7[a,b]	3.5
Non-European countries		
Northern Iran: North-east Gonbad	515.6	1.1
North-west Gilan	48.7	3.5
Northern China: North-east Honan	236.6	1.6
Northern Shansi	3.9	2.3

[a] Estimate from mortality data.

[b] Estimate from a different age group.

[c] Incidence based on fewer than 10 cases.

Source: Cook-Mozaffari *(15)*.

Table 8. Incidence of registered cases of cancer per 100 000 population. USSR

Site	1965 Males	1965 Females	1970 Males	1970 Females	1975 Males	1975 Female	1980 Male	1980 Females
Lip	13.6	2.0	12.1	1.7	10.8	1.6	9.5	1.4
Oesophagus	11.7	5.1	10.8	4.6	9.4	3.9	8.7	3.3
Stomach	62.1	33.4	57.4	28.9	53.9	25.3	47.2	21.0
Rectum	3.6	3.5	4.7	4.3	6.3	5.3	7.8	6.1
Bronchus, trachea	37.7	5.6	43.2	6.1	49.3	7.1	55.0	7.1
Skin	19.1	18.5	19.3	18.2	20.9	18.9	21.2	18.5
Haemopoetic and lymphatic tissue	6.3	4.0	8.9	5.8	10.3	6.6	10.4	6.8
Breast		13.7		15.2		19.2		22.2
Cervix uteri		26.2		21.4		18.7		16.2
All sites	199.2	144.6	207.8	143.1	220.3	148.0	225.3	147.8

Note. Figures are age-standardized (using the standard population of Segi; USSR in 1966) annual registration rates per 100 000 population for the whole of the USSR.

Source: Napalkov et al., ed. *(16)*.

Table 9. Gastric cancer mortality rate for males
per 100 000 population standardized to the "world population"

Country	1961	1971	1981–1984
Belgium	30.6	22.7	13.4[a]
Czechoslovkia	44.8	36.0	24.3[b]
Denmark	24.6	16.2	10.4[c]
Finland	44.1	29.8	16.9[d]
France	25.0	16.9	12.1[b]
Germany, Federal Republic of	39.6	30.0	19.7[c]
Greece	15.6	13.5	10.8[b]
Hungary	45.5	39.7	29.5[c]
Iceland	63.6	34.2	23.6[d]
Ireland	24.2	22.1	15.0[b]
Israel (Jewish population)	19.7	17.3	10.0[d]
Italy	34.1	30.0	21.8[b]
Netherlands	31.1	22.8	16.4[c]
Norway	29.4	21.1	14.5[c]
Poland	41.3	38.2	27.2[a]
Portugal	31.8	36.9	27.9[c]
Sweden	25.6	17.3	12.4[b]
Switzerland	31.5	22.1	11.5[a]
United Kingdom: England & Wales	25.3	20.8	15.2[c]
Northern Ireland	25.9	20.9	15.3[b]
Scotland	27.9	22.9	14.6[d]
Yugoslavia	22.3	22.4	20.7[b]

[a] Figure from 1984.

[b] Figure from 1981.

[c] Figure from 1982.

[d] Figure from 1983.

Source: Tulinius *(17)* and *World health statistics annual.*

communities. Incidence is higher in towns. In almost all areas, men have a
higher incidence of colon cancer than women. Similar differences occur in
the incidence of rectal cancer. The differences between urban and rural areas
are highlighted by a recent IARC study that looked at the patterns of both
diet and cancer of the large bowel in Denmark and Finland. Table 10 shows
data collected by IARC on age-standardized incidence rates in men in four
areas in Denmark and Finland. The table shows nearly a fourfold difference
in the incidence of colon cancer between rural Finland and Copenhagen. A
threefold variation in incidence rates across a single country is shown for

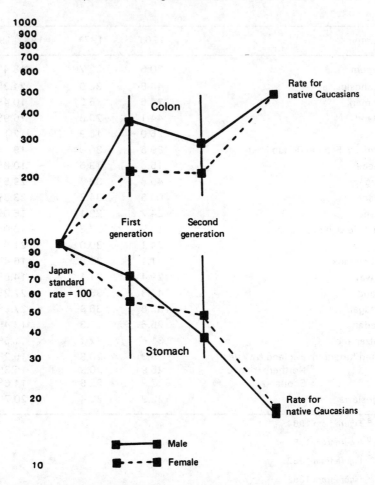

Fig. 18. Mortality from cancer of the stomach and colon in Japanese immigrants to the United States

Source: Wynder et al. *(18).*

the USSR in Fig. 19. The standard data reporting system allows only for the collection of data on rectal cancer, as defined in category 154.1 of the ninth revision of the ICD. This excludes the rectosigmoid junction and the anal canal. In both men and women, the highest rates are observed in the Baltic republics. These rates are similar to those of other European registries although, in both men and women, they increased over the period 1965–1980. In addition, although all these regions are within the USSR and are therefore considered by the Regional Office for Europe, many of them are in the Asian part of the country.

Table 10. Colon and rectal cancer: average annual age-standardized incidence rates[a] per 100 000 population among men in four areas surveyed in Denmark and Finland

| Country (period) | Study area | Incidence rates | | |
		Colon	Rectum	Total
Finland (1970–1975)	Parikkala (rural)	6.7	7.5	14.2
	Helsinki	17.0	8.7	25.7
Denmark (1968–1972)	Them (rural)	12.9	15.0	27.9
	Copenhagen	22.8	19.3	42.1

[a] These rates are standardized to the "world population structure".

Source: Jensen *(19)*.

Fig. 19. Incidence of rectal cancer per 100 000 population in regions of the USSR

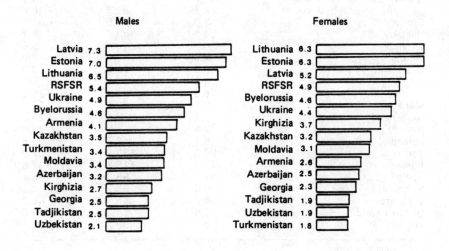

Males

Latvia 7.3
Estonia 7.0
Lithuania 6.5
RSFSR 5.4
Ukraine 4.9
Byelorussia 4.6
Armenia 4.1
Kazakhstan 3.5
Turkmenistan 3.4
Moldavia 3.4
Azerbaijan 3.2
Kirghizia 2.7
Georgia 2.5
Tadjikistan 2.5
Uzbekistan 2.1

Females

Lithuania 6.3
Estonia 6.3
Latvia 5.2
RSFSR 4.9
Byelorussia 4.6
Ukraine 4.4
Kirghizia 3.7
Kazakhstan 3.2
Moldavia 3.1
Armenia 2.6
Azerbaijan 2.5
Georgia 2.3
Tadjikistan 1.9
Uzbekistan 1.9
Turkmenistan 1.8

Source: Waterhouse et al. *(20)*.

Cirrhosis of the liver

As with other diseases, the rates of death from cirrhosis of the liver vary remarkably among and within countries (Table 11 and Fig. 20).

In Italy, as elsewhere, men clearly have a higher incidence of cirrhosis than women, but the pattern of the disease around the country is not consistent in the two sexes. Thus, the high incidence in women in the Naples area does not correspond to a similar very high rate in men. Women are

Table 11. Mortality rates from cirrhosis of the liver
per 100 000 population, males,
five-year averages over the period 1980–1984

Country	Age group (years)		
	35–39	55–59	75–79
Austria	19.4	120.1	152.6
Belgium	8.0	38.4	66.1
Bulgaria	6.8	47.5	69.5
Czechoslovakia	20.3	78.2	111.3
Denmark	11.1	44.1	38.0
Finland	7.1	28.2	24.4
France	11.8	109.3	138.2
German Democratic Republic[a]	11.5	51.3	78.7
Germany, Federal Republic of	18.3	81.6	135.6
Greece	2.8	33.9	83.9
Hungary	31.3	133.7	135.7
Iceland	0.0	0.0	0.0
Ireland[b]	2.0	9.6	17.0
Israel	3.0	28.4	50.5
Italy[c]	14.6	118.0	216.6
Luxembourg	16.5	81.4	125.0
Malta	3.2	52.6	57.4
Netherlands	3.2	17.6	25.7
Norway	2.4	16.8	21.0
Poland	5.1	42.6	92.5
Portugal	20.9	132.5	167.9
Romania	16.1	116.8	163.8
Spain[d]	11.7	98.3	135.1
Sweden	6.6	35.2	30.7
Switzerland	5.2	45.0	88.7
United Kingdom	2.8	14.2	14.6
Yugoslavia[e]	15.5	99.1	122.3

[a] Data from 1984.

[b] Data from 1980–1983.

[c] Data from 1980–1981.

[d] Data from 1980.

[e] Data from 1980–1982.

Fig. 20. Incidence of cirrhosis of the liver per 100 000 population. Italy. 1979

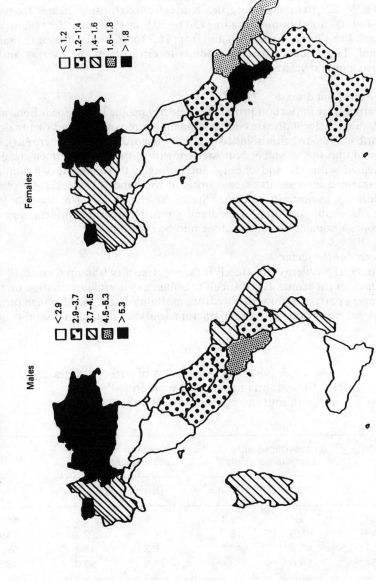

Males

☐	<2.9
	2.9–3.7
▨	3.7–4.5
▨	4.5–5.3
■	>5.3

Females

☐	<1.2
	1.2–1.4
▨	1.4–1.6
▨	1.6–1.8
■	>1.8

Source: La mortalità in Italia. 1970–79 (21).

41

considered to be particularly susceptible to cirrhosis in areas where alcohol consumption is high, but other factors such as hepatitis also operate.

Rates of mortality from cirrhosis may change rapidly. For example, during the First World War, when alcohol consumption fell precipitately, the mortality rate from cirrhosis of the liver also fell markedly. In the last 25 years the death rates have, in general, doubled in most European countries, although they fell in France, Spain and Switzerland between 1971 and 1974 (22). In Luxembourg, death rates from cirrhosis increased from 9.4 per 100 000 adult population in 1950 to 30.9 in 1975; and they increased from 2.4 to 17.6 in Yugoslavia and from 16.7 to 42.5 in Italy over the same period. The evidence therefore points to cirrhosis of the liver as an increasing public health problem.

Bone and joint disease

A particularly important problem for elderly people in Europe is bone and joint disease. Joint disease comprises mainly osteoarthritis and rheumatoid arthritis. Osteoarthritis is linked to obesity, according to Silberberg (23). He showed that the prevalence of osteoarthritis of the feet in women steadily increased with age and obesity. Interestingly, there was also a similar, unexplained increase in osteoarthritis of the hands (Table 12). Of obese middle-aged women in the United States, 50% have osteoarthritis of the feet and 73.4% abnormalities of the hand joints. Comparable information on European populations does not seem to be available.

Fracture of the femur

A principal problem in the elderly is the occurrence of fractures, especially in the neck of the femur. It is difficult to obtain any useful information on the changing pattern of bone disease from mortality statistics. Although proximal fracture of the femur, or hip fracture, leads to substantial disability and

Table 12. Increasing prevalence of osteoarthritis of
the hands and feet of women with age
and with increasing amounts of subcutaneous fat

Age (years)	Osteoarthritis of hands: subscapular skinfold		Osteoarthritis of feet: subscapular skinfold		No. of women studied
	1–10 mm	31–65 mm	1–10 mm	31–65 mm	
25–34	1.4	7.1	3.1	9.5	667
35–44	6.5	15.9	8.3	12.2	748
45–54	17.8	40.0	16.3	34.7	697
55–64	56.0	73.4	22.0	50.0	436

Source: Engel (24).

elderly patients may die from pneumonia following surgery, the primary event leading to death may not be recorded and many patients survive surgery. Incidence figures are therefore a much more useful indicator of the extent of the problem. There is some evidence that the pattern of bone disease varies across Europe and that the problem is increasing. Increases have been demonstrated in Oslo, Norway; Gothenburg, Malmö and Stockholm, Sweden; and in Dundee, Nottingham and Oxford, United Kingdom. Mannius et al. *(25)* presented evidence on differences between urban and rural areas and noted that in the county of Skaraborg, 100–150 km from Gothenburg, the annual incidence of fracture of the femur has also risen rapidly, although the rate is lower among the rural population. The increase in Gothenburg is of long standing, with rising numbers of cases being observed from about 1950.

An example of the changing pattern is shown in Table 13. The incidence rate has increased greatly with age in this British population. In the last 30 years, the rate has doubled, even when allowance is made for demographic changes. There is thus a true increase in incidence as well as an increase in the number of the elderly. The implications of these demographic changes should not be underestimated; fracture of the femur is becoming a major problem, leading to substantial morbidity and requiring sophisticated hospital care and substantial resources for surgery and rehabilitation. The work of Boyce & Vessey *(26)* is reinforced by a number of studies that show a long-term true increase in the incidence rate of fracture of the proximal femur in the United Kingdom. Within any one country, however, the changing rates can be surprisingly different. For example, in the southwest region of Great Britain, the number of people admitted to hospital with fracture of the femur doubled in only 10 years, while admissions in the Oxford area increased by only 18%. Environmental factors rather than changes in the age structure may be responsible for these differences.

Table 13. Annual age-specific incidence per 10 000 population
for fracture of the proximal femur
in people over the age of 34 years in Oxford, United Kingdom

Age (years)	Males		Females	
	1954–1958	1983	1954–1958	1983
35–54	1.1	2.1	1.1	1.9
55–64	6.5	6.3	4.0	9.3
65–74	6.7	11.6	15.3	21.6
75–84	21.8	53.1	52.6	111.8
≧ 85	48.8	131.6	140.5	322.3

Source: Boyce & Vessey *(26)*.

The progressive increase in the incidence of fracture of the femur in Sweden may have ceased, having previously been about 10% per year *(27)*.[a] Incidence in men of all ages seemed to have increased more rapidly than in women. In Sweden, hip fractures account for an annual death rate of about 40 per 100 000 population in divorced men of 70–74 years; the rate is only 15 per 100 000 in married men of the same age. Men's social pattern and lifestyle seem to be important factors. In part, this difference may be attributable to the higher level of smoking among divorced men since the mineral content of elderly people's bones is inversely related to cigarette smoking. The mineral content of smokers' bones is 15–30% lower than that of nonsmokers.[a]

Oral disease

The two major oral diseases, periodontal disease and dental caries, are major problems in Europe and in all western societies.

Periodontal disease is any disease peculiar to the tissues surrounding the teeth. The common form usually begins in childhood as inflammation of the gum margin, leading to swelling and bleeding of the gums when the teeth are brushed; this stage is classified as gingivitis. This condition gradually leads to chronic periodontitis when the bone and fibres below the gum are progressively attacked, leading eventually to the loosening and then loss of the tooth. The problem is widespread in Europe.

The initial lesion of the gum and its subsequent progression is strongly associated with bacterial plaque at or beneath the gum margin. The severity of the disease is affected not only by the extent of the plaque but also by the degree to which the gums react to the products of bacterial fermentation below the plaque. As the disease progresses, plaque accumulates in a periodontal pocket formed by the widening of the small gap between the gum margin and the tooth. The reasons for the wide variation in the rate of destruction of the bone that supports the teeth are unknown, however, although both hormonal and metabolic factors are involved. For example, the gums of pregnant women have an exaggerated response to plaque.

Dental caries, or tooth decay, is so widespread in most European countries as to be an established feature of life. Over 90% of children aged 15 years have some decay; our ancestors suffered far less from this condition. More recently, the prevalence of dental caries has begun to decline, probably in response to the widespread introduction of fluoride in toothpaste, in treatment of children's teeth, and in the public water supply in many countries. In addition, oral hygiene has improved. The prevalence of dental caries in children in 47 countries is shown in Fig. 21. Because dental caries is so widespread and leads to pain and tooth loss if left untreated, effective control can only be achieved through prevention. This is, fortunnately, quite possible.

---

[a] **Mellström, D. & Rundgren, A.** *Aspects of the pathogenesis and consequences of osteoporosis.* Copenhagen, WHO Regional Office for Europe, 1984 (unpublished document ICP/NUT 102/m01/7).

Fig. 21. Prevalence of dental decay, expressed as decayed, missing and filled teeth (DMFT) in children aged 12 years, and per capita daily sugar supply in 47 countries

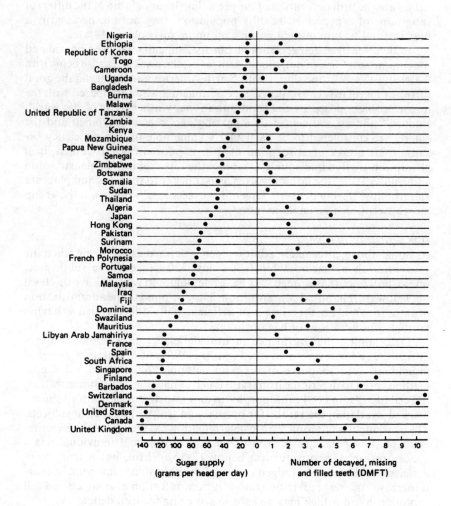

Sugar supply
(grams per head per day)

Number of decayed, missing
and filled teeth (DMFT)

Source: Sreebny *(28).*

45

Anaemia

The criteria for diagnosing anaemia were set nearly 30 years ago by WHO with the arbitrary choice of certain haemoglobin concentrations as cut-off points. Subsequently, the limits of normality were changed, with children aged from 6 months to 6 years and pregnant women having a lower normal limit of haemoglobin (110 g/litre), older children aged 5–18 years and nonpregnant women 120 g/litre, and adult males 130 g/litre *(29)*. The values are the fifth percentiles of the prevailing haemoglobin of the different subgroups of a presumed healthy population; they are not necessarily a fundamental feature of each group's optimum physiological state.

In the industrialized societies of Europe, anaemia has been considered the commonest form of nutritional deficiency, the principal cause being iron deficiency. Yet Europe shares with North America and Australia the good fortune of a relatively low prevalence of anaemia when compared with the major problem posed by the condition in many other parts of the world. Infants, children, women of childbearing age, pregnant women and the elderly are considered to be particularly vulnerable to iron deficiency because their intake or absorption of iron is poor. In adult women, iron absorption is often inadequate to replace the losses of iron in menstruation and childbearing; the latter involves iron transfer to the fetus and placenta and iron loss during delivery. Given this excess loss, women are the group most susceptible to iron deficiency.

Iron deficiency in women

As noted above, anaemia in adult women is defined as occurring when the concentration of haemoglobin falls below 120 g/litre. More subtle tests reveal, however, that women may have haemoglobin values above this level but below their habitual concentration. They respond to the administration of extra iron and are therefore iron-deficient while still classified as having normal concentrations of haemoglobin.

Determining the prevalence of iron deficiency in a population is a difficult task for several reasons. First, it is difficult to obtain a group of individuals representative of the whole population. Second, all simple methods used to determine iron status (such as haemoglobin concentration, red cell indices, red cell protoporphyrin and transferrin saturation) show a marked overlap in the results for normal and truly iron-deficient subjects. The introduction of serum ferritin determination has facilitated the measurement of the prevalence of iron deficiency. No normal individual has a concentration of serum ferritin below 12–15 μg/litre, but a truly iron-deficient woman may be judged normal if she has a minor infection because it increases the serum ferritin concentration. Infection also affects red cell protoporphyrin, which may be used in screening for iron deficiency.

Comparative studies on the prevalence of iron deficiency in different populations depend mainly on assessing the prevalence of anaemia. Of course, the extent of the overlap in the distribution curves of the haemoglobin values in normal and iron-deficient women is not the same in all populations. In developing countries, where more frequent and severe iron-deficiency anaemia occurs, the overlap is much less marked than in developed countries.

In a study in Gothenburg *(30)* of a random sample of 38-year-old women in 1968, only 5.4% had haemoglobin values below 120 g/litre. However, 31% had no iron stores; visible iron was absent from the reticulo-endothelial cells of the bone marrow. This method of testing, carefully undertaken with technically adequate smears, is generally considered the best way to determine iron deficiency. It is therefore the basis for evaluating other methods. In the Gothenburg study, measurements of serum ferritin showed that about 30% of the women had subnormal ferritin levels and therefore had potential iron deficiency. Oral iron supplementation revealed that about 30% of these women were true responders. Therefore, while about 10% of the women had no iron stores and suboptimum haemoglobin levels, only 5.4% of the sample met the criteria for anaemia. This indicates that the use of haemoglobin tests as the only indicator of iron-deficiency anaemia diagnoses about half of those with true iron deficiency.

In a new sample of 38-year-old women in Gothenburg *(31)* examined in 1980, the prevalence of anaemia had increased to 7.4%; 29.5% still had subnormal serum ferritin values. This figure implies that an appreciable minority of adult women in Sweden still have iron deficiency. Other Scandinavian studies, made in Denmark *(32–34)*, Norway *(35,36)* and Finland *(37)*, provide population data. They all show a prevalence of anaemia of about 5%. None of a group of Danish blood donors *(34)* had anaemia according to the WHO definition, but 22.1% had subnormal serum ferritin levels. Since it is reasonable to assume that women with a history of anaemia are less likely to volunteer as blood donors, the true prevalence of iron deficiency will be underestimated if reliance is placed on the data collected from blood donors. One study *(36)* shows a prevalence of anaemia in England similar to that in Scandinavia; it also shows that about 30% of women of childbearing age have iron deficiency. The results of these studies are summarized in Table 14.

The non-random French sample *(38)* showed a lower prevalence of both anaemia (1.3%) and iron deficiency (16%) and a random sample of German women in Heidelberg *(39)* had a prevalence of anaemia of only 2.4% (Table 14). In the USSR, however, 9% had overt anaemia and 18% latent iron deficiency *(40)*. The prevalence of iron deficiency probably varies among regions in Europe.

Pregnancy
Concentrations of haemoglobin in pregnant women usually decline because of the increase in their blood volume and therefore in the demand for iron to provide additional haemoglobin in the expanded red cell mass. For example, if a woman normally has a haemoglobin concentration of 135 g/litre and a blood volume of 4 litres, she has a total circulating haemoglobin mass of about 540 g. If she becomes pregnant and her haemoglobin drops to 100 g/litre by the end of her pregnancy, her total haemoglobin will still have increased to 580 g because her blood volume is now 5.4 litres. The use of iron supplements during pregnancy can prevent much of the fall in haemoglobin *(41)*, but, even in women taking extra oral iron in adequate amounts, haemoglobin decreases slightly as the increase in plasma volume exceeds the

Table 14. Prevalence of iron deficiency in women in different European areas

Country and area	Year of study	Age of subjects (years)	No. of subjects	Percentage of women with:		
				anaemia (haemoglobin <120 g/litre)	subnormal serum ferritin level	absence of stainable bone marrow iron
Sweden: Gothenburg	1968	38	372	5.4	~30	31.0
	1980	38	122	7.4	29.5	
Denmark:						
Fyn	1977	15–24	997	4.3		
Glostrup	1976	40	548	5.0		
First-time blood donors	1981	18–45	163	0.0	22.1	
Norway	1973	17–50	64	12.5		
	1976	≧17	208	5.8		
Finland: whole country	1966–1972	15–19	2616	3.6		
		20–29	3827	3.9		
		30–39	3431	6.5		
		40–49	3632	11.0		
England & Wales	1966	≧18	} 465, 393	6.5, 7.4		31.0
France: Paris	1985	17–42	476	1.3	16.2	
Germany, Federal Republic of: Heidelberg	1978–1979	20–40	553	2.4		

rise in red cell mass. The physiological anaemia of pregnancy amounts to a fall of 10–20 g/litre haemoglobin. Levels of iron are difficult to interpret in pregnancy. Iron levels in plasma tend to decline by about 35%, transferrin concentrations increase, and transferrin saturation is markedly reduced in a manner unrelated to iron stores *(42)*. Red cell protoporphyrin increases to a small degree but serum ferritin falls remarkably; even with iron supplements, a group of women in the second half of pregnancy may have an average serum ferritin level of only 15 µg/litre, the cut-off point for diagnosing iron deficiency *(43)*.

These observations have led to much debate about an appropriate policy on iron supplements in pregnancy. The total amount of iron that needs to be absorbed in the last trimester of pregnancy is very high and may reach 8–10 mg per day. No diet can provide such large amounts of absorbed iron, so iron requirements in pregnancy can only be met by drawing on the body's iron stores. At least 500 mg of stored iron is needed at the start of pregnancy. The diet of our ancestors probably allowed a woman to build up sufficiently large iron stores before her first pregnancy. Prolonged lactation and a good diet probably allowed a restitution of iron stores between pregnancies. The present approach of routinely recommending extra oral iron to all pregnant women should be considered in such a perspective. In some countries, the routine provision of oral iron to pregnant women, regardless of their hae-moglobin level is tending to be replaced by a more specific policy of routinely providing iron after birth or providing it during pregnancy when there is clear evidence of iron deficiency (a haemoglobin concentration below 100 g/litre with a mean corpuscular volume of under 82 femtolitres). The problems of managing anaemia will clearly be reduced if women start pregnancy with adequate iron stores, and the use of supplements may be the more appropriate preventive policy.

Children and adolescents
Babies initially have low iron stores, particularly if they have been breastfed for several months and therefore rely predominantly on the iron already stored at birth. Premature babies, with very low iron stores, are therefore particularly vulnerable to anaemia.

Iron is a component of tissue enzymes and proteins as well as circulating haemoglobin. As children grow, they therefore have a great need for iron. Below the age of one year and from 6 to 16 years of age, children need as much or more iron than adults. Since they are smaller and require less energy than adults, the amount of iron absorbed per unit of dietary energy must be substantially more than in adult life. After menarche, girls need to replace menstrual losses of iron in addition to meeting the heavy demands for iron for tissue growth, although individuals' needs may vary widely. It is therefore not surprising that nutritionists and physicians have paid par-ticular attention to nutritional anaemia in childhood.

In many European populations, the overall prevalence of anaemia can be expected to be about 5% (as implied by the choice of the fifth percentile in defining anaemia), but the majority of anaemic children come from families with low socioeconomic status. In a Bulgarian study of children aged 1–3 years *(44)*, 11.5% of the children had a haemoglobin level below 94 g/litre and 62% were considered to have low concentrations of serum iron (<600 µg/litre). Most of these children were looked after in crèches during the day.

Variations in the prevalence of anaemia are also found within countries. For example, 2.6–4.1% of Warsaw adolescents aged 10–18 years had anaemia on the basis of the WHO classification, compared with 9.7–11.4% of those in the Ciechanow area *(45)*. In addition, while serum ferritin values were below 10 µg/litre in 18.5% of healthy children aged from 6 months to 3 years in Budapest, 41% of comparable Hungarian children living in the county of Borsod had low values. Educational status was one indication of the poorer socioeconomic conditions in the less affluent county, but a comparable study of Hungarian gypsies *(46)* showed no children with low serum ferritin despite the families' supposedly lower purchasing power. Thus, iron deficiency is not necessarily directly correlated with socio-economic conditions.

The elderly

Assessing the prevalence of iron deficiency and anaemia in elderly people is difficult because haemoglobin concentrations appear to decline slowly and progressively with age for reasons that remain obscure. The prevalence of true anaemia is therefore more likely to be overestimated in the older age groups.

Some systematic studies of anaemia have been undertaken in the elderly population of some European countries. In the Dalby survey in Sweden *(47)*, a small number of men and women aged 67–73 years were examined at intervals from 1969 to 1975. Three of the 17 men had haemoglobin concentrations below 130 g/litre on one of the four examinations; three of the 20 women had concentrations below 120 g/litre at some time during the study. In the United Kingdom, a more extensive survey of 879 men and women aged over 65 years diagnosed 16.9% of the men and 8.8% of the women as having anaemia *(48)*. Subnormal values for serum iron and total iron-binding capacity were taken to reflect iron deficiency; 19.3% of the men and 24.6% of the women had such low values. Iron deficiency thus seems to be very common in the elderly. A French study *(49)* found a 20% prevalence of anaemia in elderly people in hospitals and in homes for the aged.

Folic acid deficiency

This deficiency is an uncommon cause of anaemia in European children and adults, although biochemical tests for suboptimum folic acid status may reveal an appreciable number of women with mild deficiency. This deficiency is exacerbated by the increased demands for folacin in pregnancy. In Europe, if pregnant women do not receive extra folic acid, about 30% show clear-cut signs of folic acid deficiency: changes in the red cells in the bone marrow. These changes signify inadequate folic acid supplies for tissues; they can be largely prevented by a diet rich in folic acid.

Interest in the levels of folic acid in pregnant women has recently been stimulated by the claim that an inadequate vitamin status at the time of conception leads to congenital malformation of the fetus with an increased incidence of spina bifida *(50)*. In addition, Lawrence and his colleagues in the United Kingdom assessed the diets of women who had children with neural tube defects and inferred from questionnaires that their diet was nutritionally inadequate before pregnancy *(51)*. The same authors provided 2 mg folic acid twice daily or a placebo to mothers who had previously had children with neural tube defects and were contemplating a further pregnancy. In both these studies *(50,51)*, which involved the use of supplements containing a large number of vitamins, women who received and took the folic acid or vitamins had a recurrence rate of neural tube defects in their babies of 0–1%, compared with 4.7–9% in the unsupplemented groups. The Medical Research Council in the United Kingdom is conducting a formal double-blind trial to assess the validity of these findings and to see whether a deficiency of folic acid or other vitamins is the key to the development of this congenital malformation. If this difficult study confirms Smithells' early findings, it will be of considerable importance to public health.

Effects of anaemia and iron deficiency

The possible deleterious effects of iron deficiency have been much debated. It has even been suggested that anaemia may be beneficial, as there is a statistically significant relationship between the level of haemoglobin and mortality in many affluent societies. This can be explained in part by the higher haemoglobin concentrations in smokers and in patients with chronic bronchitis, hypertension and heart disease. Users of some drugs, such as diuretics, also have higher concentrations, but the conditions for which the drugs are taken may be the real reason for the greater mortality. Recent data, however, suggest that iron deficiency is a problem since it may limit work capacity and leads to apathy, irritability, impaired attentiveness and reduced learning ability in children. If these functional effects prove to be proportional to the degree of iron deficiency, even modest reductions in haemoglobin must be considered disadvantageous. Immunological abnormalities have also been demonstrated in iron deficiency, but their clinical relevance remains uncertain.

Nutritionists often define the minimum requirement of a vitamin or mineral as an amount that does not simply avoid a clinical deficiency but allows the body to build up stores adequate to buffer temporary increases in need or a fall in intake. On this basis, children and adults without any iron reserves may reasonably be considered to need more iron; current evidence implies that sufficient dietary iron is required to maintain iron stores and that these can be monitored indirectly by measuring circulating serum ferritin concentrations. A normal value of above $15\,\mu g/$litre for serum ferritin would seem to be a reasonable criterion for adequate iron intake.

Goitre

Goitre was one of the most important nutritional deficiency diseases of Europe until major efforts were made to increase iodine intakes after the Second World War. A comprehensive review of the current position has recently been published *(52)*. The prevalence of goitre is not the only index

Table 15. Goitre and iodine deficiency and prophylaxis in Europe

Group and country	Prevalence of goitre[a]	Iodine intake[b]	Iodine prophylaxis[c]
No endemic goitre			
Denmark	0	b/s	n
Finland	0	s	m
Iceland	0?	s	–
Ireland	0/1	s	v
Norway	0	s	v
Sweden	0	s	m
United Kingdom	0/1	s	n
Intermediate			
Belgium	0/1	b	v
Bulgaria	1	s	m
Czechoslovakia	1	s	m
Netherlands	1	s	m
Switzerland	1	s	m
Endemic goitre			
Iodine prophylaxis mandatory			
Austria	2	b	m
Hungary	2	b	m
Poland	2	b	m
Yugoslavia	2	b	m
Iodine prophylaxis not mandatory			
German Democratic Republic	2	i	v
Germany, Federal Republic of	2	i	v
Greece	2	i	v
Italy	2(3)	i	v
Portugal	2(3)	i	v
Romania	2	b	–
Spain	2(3)	i	v
Turkey	2	i	v
Information unobtainable			
Albania	–	–	–
France	1?	b	v
USSR	1?	–	–

[a] 0 = practically none; 1 = < 10%; 2 = 10–30% (or more); 3 = risk of endemic cretinism; – = no information.

[b] s = sufficient; b = borderline sufficient; i = insufficient; – = no information.

[c] m = mandatory (or v > 90%); v = voluntary; n = none; – = no information.

Source: European Thyroid Association *(52)*.

of iodine deficiency in a community, however, and one of the principal concerns in iodine deficiency is the prevention of cretinism and the milder forms of retardation that Hetzel has called collectively the iodine deficiency disorders *(53)*.

Table 15 classifies the countries of Europe according to whether goitre is prevalent and whether iodine prophylaxis is mandatory. The northern countries and the United Kingdom have no endemic goitre, but other European countries are not so fortunate.

The intermediate group comprises four countries that have had major problems with endemic goitre in the past but have introduced effective prevention programmes. Iodine intake is now adequate. Epidemiological surveys have shown that goitre persists in some adults in these countries but that it is seldom seen in children. Belgium probably belongs in this group because iodine prophylaxis is voluntary and urine iodine excretion studies indicate that iodine intake is not adequate in all regions. These data, however, are incomplete, and further surveys are required.

It is disturbing that 12 countries (50% of those surveyed) make up a group in which endemic goitre persists.

Four countries make up a subgroup in which iodine prophylaxis is mandatory, although substantial areas of high goitre prevalence nevertheless persist. Dietary iodine intake remains borderline, and the analysis of the iodine content of salt from three of these countries gave values of 4–12 mg/kg.

In the large subgroup in which iodine prophylaxis is not mandatory, goitre continues to be a major problem, either nationally or regionally, and iodine intakes are so low in some regions that the risk of cretinism persists. Iodine prophylaxis programmes are urgently required. In these countries and elsewhere, health policy-makers need to consider how best to provide additional iodine when the use of salt in the home is discouraged as part of a policy to reduce the prevalence of high blood pressure.

3

Conditions predisposing to major health problems

Obesity

Obesity has been recognized as a nutritional problem in Europe, as well as in other countries, but no systematic assessment has been made of the variation in its prevalence in different countries. The choice of a definition of obesity is important. At the First International Conference on Body Weight Control *(54)*, it was agreed that a simple definition of ideal or optimum weight should be a body mass index (BMI, weight in kg divided by (height in metres)^2) of 20–25. This conforms with the earlier recommendations of the Fogarty Conference *(55)* in the United States and of the British Royal College of Physicians *(56)*.

Overweight can then be classified as a BMI in excess of 25 (grade 1 obesity). Above a BMI of 30, people can be described as having classical obesity (grade 2 obesity), and Garrow *(57)* has suggested a third grade of obesity for people with a BMI over 40. This approach has not as yet been universally applied. Many European studies employ the more complicated Broca index, in which normal weight (in kg) is defined as equal to height (in cm) minus 100; obesity occurs when the weight is 20% in excess of this value. In practice, this gives a normal Broca weight within the BMI range of 20 to 25, lower values being found in short people. Bearing these differences in mind and defining overweight as a BMI of 25–30, it is interesting to compare data on the prevalence of overweight and obesity in different individual surveys throughout Europe (Table 16), as collated by Kluthe & Schubert *(58)*. These data range in time from studies conducted shortly after the Second World War to those performed since 1980. The table summarizes evidence of a higher prevalence of obesity in women in four countries. A survey in Italy *(59)* showed that the majority of middle-aged Italians were overweight and about 10% of men and 15% of women had grade 2 obesity (Table 17).

In 1981, a more comprehensive survey in Great Britain *(60)* also found that women were more frankly obese (grades 2 and 3) than men but less overweight (grade 1). Prevalence changed with age. Women tended to be more overweight later in middle age, and by the age of 60–64 years, 49% of British women had a BMI higher than 25. Similar figures are also available

Table 16. Prevalence of obesity in Europe

Country and study population	Age (years)	No. of subjects	Obesity index	Prevalence (%)		
				Males	Females	Both
Austria						
Health check-up	20–40	...	>20% over Broca[a]	13.7–27	17.6–41	5–15
	60		>20% over Broca			...
Bulgaria						
83% of nine villages	35–≧74	4198	>20% over Broca	...	...	19.1
Denmark						
Military sample	18–20	551	≧25.7 BMI	9.9	...	...
Copenhagen	18–20	263	≧25.7 BMI	10.2	...	...
German Democratic Republic						
Rural sample	...	1918	>20% over Broca	16.0	41.0	...
Rural and small-town population	...	30516	>20% over Broca	27.0	52.0	...
Representative population	...	79708	>20% over Broca	...	...	...
Town	...		>20% over Broca	14.0	32.0	...
Rural	...	...	>20% over Broca	23.0	49.0	...
Germany, Federal Republic of						
Sample	...	1904	>15% over Broca	16.3	18.2	17.4
Municipalities of Eberbach, Wiesloch	30–60	4709	>20% over Broca	14.0	...	...
Life insurance contracts, 1955	...	...	>40% over Broca	...	...	8.0
Great Britain						
National representative cohort	20–26	5362	>20% over Broca	5–12	6–11	...

	Age	n			
Netherlands					
Young adults in Ede	19–31	3857	25.0–29.9 BMI	22	12
			≧30.0 BMI	2	2
Norway					
Twenty industrial physicians' offices, Oslo	40–49	3751	>15–25% over Broca	14.1	: :
Romania					
	15–65	100482	>20% over MLI[b]	: :	: :
Town	15–65	: :	>20% over MLI	25.4	32.2
Rural	15–65	: :	>20% over MLI	22.2	40.9
Switzerland					
Officials in Thun and Wimmis	31–60	1014	>25% over Broca	: :	: :
	31–40	: :	>25% over Broca	18.7	: :
	41–50	: :	>25% over Broca	28.1	: :
	51–60	: :	>25% over Broca	33.6	: :
Chemical industry employees, Basle	25–34	149	≧26.4 BMI	14.5	: :
	35–44	721	≧26.4 BMI	27.5	: :
	45–54	1187	≧26.4 BMI	35.5	: :
	55–64	934	≧26.4 BMI	44.0	: :
	65	339	≧26.4 BMI	43.0	: :
Seven countries study					
Northern Europe (Finland, Netherlands)	40–59	2439	≧27 BMI	13.0	: :
Southern Europe (Italy, Greece, Yugoslavia)	40–59	6519	≧27 BMI	23.1	: :

[a] Broca normal weight.

[b] Metropolitan Life Insurance recommended weight.

Source: Kluthe & Schubert *(58)*.

Table 17. Overweight and obesity in Italy

Age group (years)	Grade 1 obesity (%)		Grade 2 obesity (%)	
	Males	Females	Males	Females
20–29	30	25	3	3
30–39	50	40	7	6
40–49	60	55	10	15
50–59	60	62	15	25

Source: Mancini et al. *(59)*.

for Norway. Waaler *(61)* based his measurements on 1.8 million Norwegians measured between 1963 and 1975 during the course of a mass radiography programme. The average BMI of different age groups in both Norway and Great Britain are shown in Fig. 22. In both populations, weight progressively increased with age in both men and women. In Great Britain, the average male in his forties was overweight, and this also applied to all older age groups *(60)*. The Norwegian values are very similar, except that older Norwegian women appear to be heavier. A similar accentuation of obesity with age is seen in Austrian women *(58)*.

The significance of obesity
These judgements on the appropriateness of weight depend on a series of analyses linking body weight to mortality and morbidity. Details have been set out by Garrow *(62)* and are based on the Build study *(63)* and a major study by Lew & Garfinkel *(64)*. The data from the second study are of great importance because, for the first time, it is possible to distinguish between the health risks of smokers and nonsmokers at various body weights. The deleterious effect of smoking is shown in Fig. 23; it is much more harmful to be a smoker of normal weight than to be a moderately obese nonsmoker. All age groups are combined in this figure to show the effect of smoking, but this tends to obscure the particularly deleterious effect of weight gain early in adult life.

Data in keeping with these conclusions were obtained by Waaler *(61)* and are summarized in Fig. 24, which shows the mortality rate at different weights for each age group. These figures are not adjusted to take account of smoking or the effects of illness on body weight. Mortality was lowest in men below the age of 50 years with a BMI of about 19–27 and in young women with a BMI of 19–25. In both sexes, however, the weight at which an age group had the lowest mortality rose progressively. For people in their seventies, the curve flattened and excess weight no longer had prognostic significance. This same phenomenon is shown in the Build study *(63)*.

58

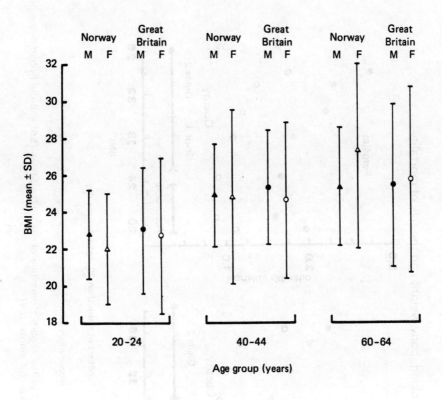

Fig. 22. BMI for males and females in Norway, 1963-1975 and Great Britain, 1981

Note. Data derived from Knight *(60)* and Waaler *(61)*.

In both the Norwegian study *(61)* and the Build study from the United States *(63)*, the demonstration of the harmful effects of excess weight is obscured because data on both smokers and nonsmokers are combined. Smokers have lower body weights but higher mortality than nonsmokers. When the data are amalgamated, the lowest mortality is therefore found at a spuriously high BMI. Additional support for the excess death rate of thin smokers comes from Waaler's analysis of death rates in relation to body weight (Fig. 25). The graphs show the percentage of the population aged 50–64 years that dies each year from eight specific conditions. Subjects who die from lung or stomach cancer or tuberculosis tend to be thin, whereas those who die from stroke or diabetes tend to be overweight. Of the people

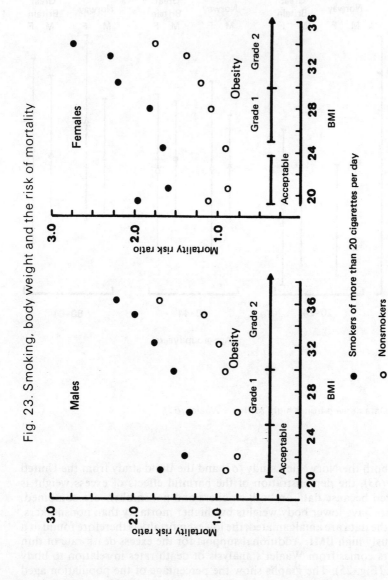

Fig. 23. Smoking, body weight and the risk of mortality

Note. Acceptable weight range is that proposed by the Fogarty Committee of the United States *(55)* and the British Royal College of Physicians *(56)*. Mortality risks recalculated from Lew & Garfinkel *(64)*.

60

Fig. 24. Mortality rates of Norwegian men and women in different age groups in relation to their BMI

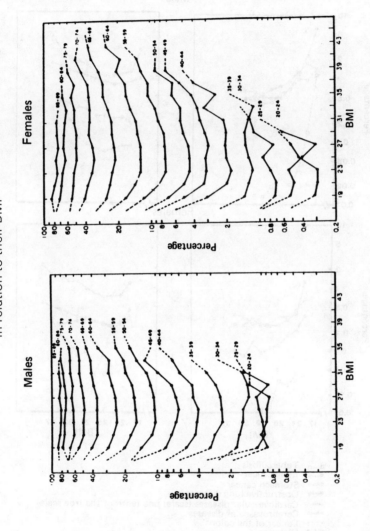

Source: Waaler (61).

Fig. 25. Mortality rates of Norwegian men and women aged 50–64 years for different diseases compared with BMI

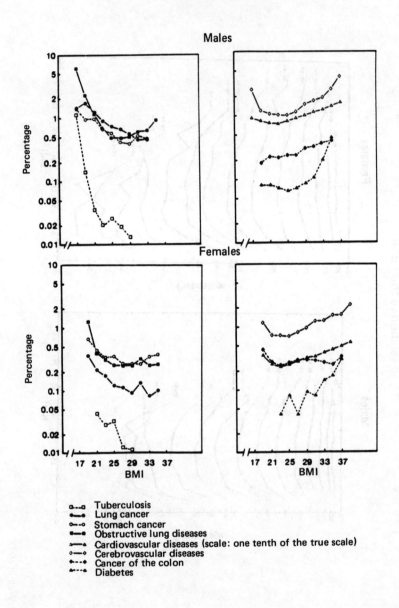

Males

Females

Tuberculosis
Lung cancer
Stomach cancer
Obstructive lung diseases
Cardiovascular diseases (scale: one tenth of the true scale)
Cerebrovascular diseases
Cancer of the colon
Diabetes

Source: Waaler *(61).*

62

aged 50–60 years, those who die of smoking-related diseases, such as obstructive lung disease and lung cancer, have much lower weights than the average. When the weights of those who die from cerbrovascular disease, cardiovascular diseases, diabetes and cancer of the colon are analysed, a very different pattern emerges; death rates increase progressively from a BMI of about 25. Note that in Fig. 25 cardiovascular deaths have been scaled down tenfold. A new analysis *(65)* linking BMI to specific causes of death (Fig. 26) also demonstrates the relationship between BMI and death from a number of diseases. Both European and American data therefore confirm that people whose weight is acceptable have a BMI of 20–25.

There has been much debate about the relationship between obesity and coronary heart disease because many investigators have found that serum cholesterol and blood pressure rise with increasing obesity. Obesity seems to increase the principal risk factors. If statistical allowance is made for the contribution of these risk factors to coronary heart disease, the independent effect of obesity proves to be very small or nonexistent. Nevertheless, in practical terms, weight reduction leads to a fall in blood pressure and can also reduce serum cholesterol. On a policy basis, therefore, it is useful to identify excess weight and obesity as a risk factor for coronary heart disease, as well as for other conditions.

More recently, it has been suggested that the distribution of fat within the body is important *(66)*. People with a paunch from excess abdominal fat and an android distribution of fat are at substantially greater risk than those with fat deposited mainly on their hips (gynaecoid distribution). This has led to the monitoring of waist and hip circumference ratios as a crude risk factor, a ratio above 0.8 indicating increased risk.

Obesity is linked not only to higher death rates but also to excess illness. Obese men and women have a greater risk of diabetes and gallstones. In adult men with a BMI of 30 or above, the incidence of diabetes increases markedly. In women, the progressive increase in the prevalence of gall-bladder disease with age is particularly marked in those who exceed the acceptable weight range *(56)*.

Obesity also increases the risk of gout, arthritis, some cancers, hernias and skin problems, as well as producing a great deal of psychological stress. The risks entailed in routine operations rise, with greater chances of venous thrombosis, chest infection and poor wound healing.

Hypertension

There are no standardized surveys of hypertension in Europe, but a new analysis is under way as part of a coordinated programme with a central data analysis centre in Heidelberg. A preliminary analysis of systolic blood pressure distributions, derived from the project on European risk factors and incidence — a collaborative analysis (ERICA) is shown in Fig. 27. The distribution curves of blood pressure are appreciably higher in northern and western Europe than in central, eastern and southern Europe *(67)*. Genetic factors influence the development of hypertension. Children whose blood pressure is in the upper quartile are much more likely to have

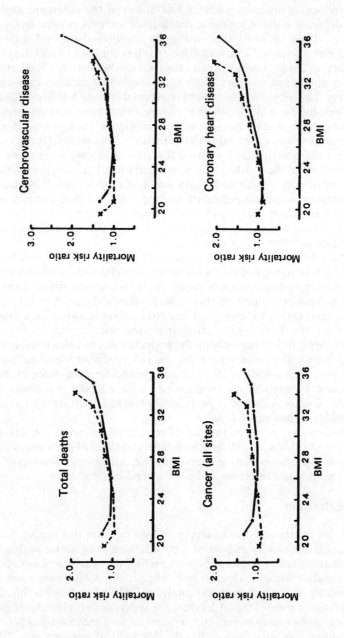

Fig. 26. The relationship between BMI and the risk of death for males and females

64

Fig. 26 (contd)

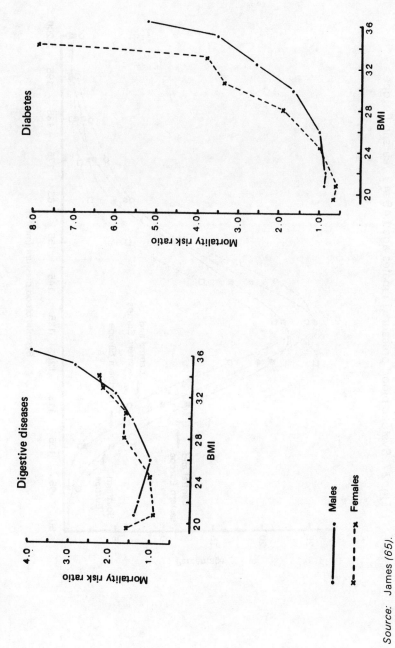

Diabetes

Digestive diseases

Males

Females

Source: James (65).

65

Fig. 27. Systolic blood pressure in males aged 45–49 years in Europe

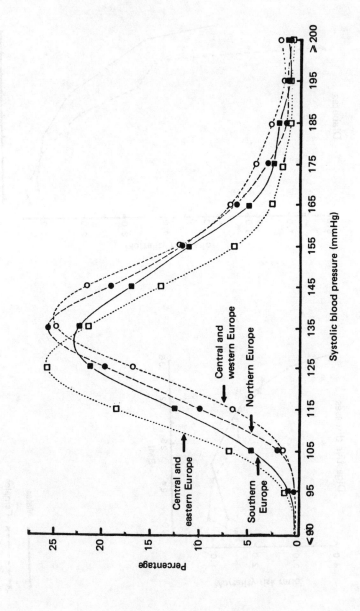

Source: Kesteloot & Van Houte (*67*).

hypertensive parents than children with low blood pressure. Children, as they grow older, also tend to maintain their blood pressure ranking within the population. Further, the upper limit for normal blood pressure is defined arbitrarily so that, with advancing years, the blood pressure of an increasing proportion of the population exceeds this limit. The progressive rise with age in the average blood pressure of the European population is striking.

As an individual factor, high blood pressure proves to be as accurate a predictor of coronary heart disease as high levels of blood sugar and cholesterol, or the number of cigarettes smoked. Fig. 28 shows how these

Fig. 28. Eight-year probability of cardiovascular disease per 1000 population, males aged 40 years, according to systolic blood pressure at specified levels of other risk factors

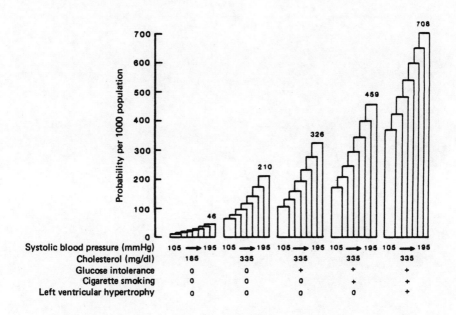

Note. The seven columns for each group of risk factors represent systolic blood pressure levels of 105, 120, 135, 150, 165, 180 and 195 mmHg.

Source: Kannel *(68).*

factors interact to increase the risk of heart disease *(68)*. Cigarette smoking amplifies the effect of hypercholesterolaemia and high blood pressure. Although men, at any level of blood pressure, have a greater absolute risk of developing coronary heart disease than women, the progressive increase in disease rates and the interaction of risk factors also apply to women.

Although blood pressure rises with age in Europe, this is not true of other regions of the world where environmental factors, including diet, are very different. The increase in blood pressure with age cannot therefore be seen as inevitable, and environmental factors must be sought. Elevated blood pressure is so common in the elderly that it is often considered to have no prognostic significance. On the contrary, high blood pressure is as much a risk factor in the elderly as in the young. It is associated with an increased risk of not only hypertensive heart disease and kidney failure but also debilitating stroke. Preventive measures for limiting this condition may therefore be as important for the elderly as for the young.

4

The role of diet in major public health problems

The secular trends in many diseases argue against genetic factors being of primary importance, and studies of migrants emphasize the crucial role of the environment. In this chapter, major public health problems are dealt with in turn and assessments are made of the degree to which diet is involved. In none of the conditions covered has a dietary factor been proved as causal, as this is exceptionally difficult, if not impossible. Supporting evidence has been obtained from cross-cultural, prospective and intervention studies, from physiological and metabolic studies in man, and from experimental studies in animals. All have been used to construct dietary hypotheses to help explain the development of a variety of health problems. National and international health policies are based on an analysis of the evidence; it must be strong enough to warrant action. Nevertheless, doubt remains about the correctness of the proposed course of action.

Coronary Heart Disease

Three principal risk factors in coronary heart disease have been identified in prospective studies throughout the world: smoking, high blood pressure and a high concentration of serum cholesterol. The risks of smoking and high serum cholesterol are discussed here, but those of hypertension are detailed in the section on cerebrovascular disease. In all societies, men have a greater risk of heart disease than women. The risk increases with age, although this increase is delayed in women until about the time of the menopause. All three of the principal risk factors are considered preventable to varying degrees, but some discussion continues about their relative importance.

Risk factors

Smoking
Smoking has been identified as a risk factor by all expert committees that have considered it. Smoking has increased substantially since the 1920s, with a marked increase following the Second World War in several countries (69). The prevalence rate of smoking varies widely, but the increase in the number of women smokers in the last 20 years has caused particular

concern. By 1980 major efforts had been made to reduce smoking rates. The countries with the most stringent antismoking policies (Norway and Poland) managed to stop the rise in tobacco sales, which in general increased by 20–50% in the last 30 years.

Fig. 29 provides evidence of a much smaller risk from smoking in some communities than in others. People in Mediterranean countries such as Greece and Italy do not appear to have a markedly increased risk of coronary heart disease despite heavy smoking (70). Indeed, France, with one of the lowest risks of coronary heart disease in Europe, has substantial tobacco consumption. These data do not imply that smoking is risk-free (since the rates of lung cancer are substantial in France, Greece and Italy) but that other factors may protect smokers from the risk. These are increasingly recognized to be dietary factors.

The pathophysiological hypothesis of Ross & Glomset (71), recently updated (72), suggests that both hypertension and smoking may act by damaging the endothelial surface of the arteries, making them in turn susceptible to damage unless appropriate repair mechanisms function. This is far less likely in people or animals with an atherogenic diet, and indeed the damage may itself precipitate further lipid accumulation. If this plausible explanation proves to be correct, then the interaction of smoking, high blood pressure and an atherogenic diet becomes clearer and a preventive policy of intervention becomes more necessary.

Smoking not only injures the arterial endothelium but also yields nicotine, which temporarily increases heart rate and blood pressure, increases myocardial oxygen demands, and lowers the threshold for abnormal cardiac rhythms. The carbon monoxide produced by smoking also leads to carboxyhaemoglobin production and a sustained decrease in the capacity of the blood to transport oxygen. In addition, smoking is a source of free radicals, increases platelet adhesiveness, and depresses concentrations of high-density lipoprotein cholesterol. All these effects can be considered likely to contribute to atherosclerosis and ischaemia of the myocardium.

Intervention trials aimed at reducing smoking rates have also been used to assess the relative importance of smoking in different communities; these will be considered later. Cigarette smoking is less consistently related to coronary heart disease in women than in men. The relationship between smoking and angina pectoris (the most common manifestation of coronary heart disease in women) is particularly weak.

Serum cholesterol

The link between the development of coronary heart disease and the level of total blood cholesterol is widely recognized. It is a good predictor of risk on a group basis in both cross-cultural studies and in cohorts within a single country.

The concentration of blood cholesterol depends on the interaction between the dietary intake of a number of nutrients and the individual's metabolic response to this diet. Intakes of saturated and polyunsaturated

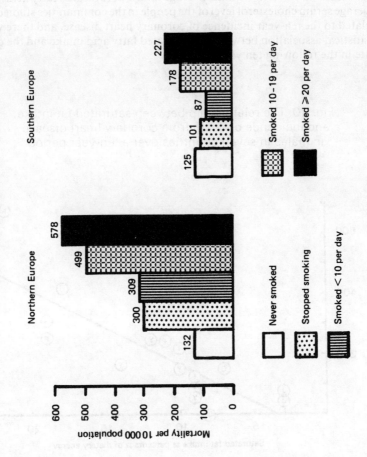

Fig. 29. Cigarette smoking and deaths from coronary heart disease per 10 000 population in northern and southern Europe

Source: Keys *(70).*

71

fatty acids are the major determinants of blood cholesterol concentration. Dietary cholesterol has a smaller effect. Both Keys et al. *(73)* and Hegstead et al. *(74)* have introduced formulae to predict changes in serum cholesterol from the intake of saturated and polyunsaturated fatty acids and of dietary cholesterol.

Keys' original study *(70)*, conducted after the Second World War, included communities in seven countries: Finland, Greece, Italy, Japan, the Netherlands, the United States and Yugoslavia. The average level of serum cholesterol had a poor relationship with total fat intake but a statistically significant association with the average intake of saturated fatty acids. The average serum cholesterol level of the people in the communities studied was related to the ten-year incidence of coronary heart disease, and there was a statistical association between the saturated fatty acid intake and the death rate in the following ten years (Fig. 30).

Fig. 30. The relationship between saturated fat intake
and incidence of death from coronary heart disease
in males in seven countries over a ten-year period

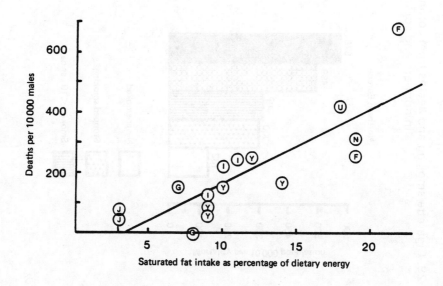

Note. F = Finland, G = Greece, I = Italy, J = Japan, N = Netherlands, U = United States, Y = Yugoslavia. The extremes in intake often apply to non-European populations.

Source: Keys *(70)*.

A number of other studies were undertaken to assess the link between diet and coronary heart disease in individuals. This individual monitoring is a difficult approach to use, since even a carefully collected, seven-day, weighed analysis of food intake, when repeated four years later on the same men, showed substantial variations in intake. The correlation coefficient for the two measurements of energy intake amounted to only $r = 0.43$ *(70)*. Predicting the habitual diet of individuals and coping with secular changes in eating habits are problems. In addition, there is also the problem of individual variability in the metabolic response to any diet. This reduces the probability of directly relating a person's saturated fatty acid intake to the risk of subsequent coronary heart disease. Overcoming some of these problems requires the study of a very large number of people. Despite these difficulties, two European studies have shown a relationship between the type of fatty acid ingested and the subsequent incidence of coronary heart disease *(75,76)*.

Since 1964, death rates in Gothenburg, Sweden from coronary heart disease have risen by 30% in men aged 50–54 years and by 20% in men aged 55–59 years *(77)*. The Gothenburg study, a longitudinal study of two groups of men born in 1913 and 1923, confirmed the importance of serum cholesterol and the other risk factors in coronary heart disease — high blood pressure and smoking — but found no significant differences between the two cohorts. Men born in 1923 were heavier and had a higher BMI than men born in 1913, indicating that men in the younger cohort tended to be more obese, but explanations for the secular increase in risk were not apparent. The increased risk occurred in spite of nationwide changes towards a more physically active lifestyle and a fall in cigarette consumption. The authors said that "a change of the diets towards consumption of fewer saturated fats and more unsaturated fats" had taken place in Sweden during the observation period *(77)*, but this does not accord with official food consumption statistics *(78)*.

The consumption of cereal fibre may also protect people against coronary heart disease for reasons that are not clear *(75)*. A fall in serum cholesterol can be produced by increasing vegetable and fruit fibre intake, but cereal fibre does not usually have this metabolic effect. The epidemiological link between coronary heart disease and the low intake of cereal fibre is therefore unexplained. In the Ireland–Boston study *(76)*, however, the people at greater risk of coronary heart disease consumed fewer vegetables. Part of the effect of a high-fibre diet, rich in cereals and vegetables, in preventing heart disease may relate to its other effects, such as the lowering of blood pressure observed when people change to a vegetarian diet. This diet has many differences from the usual mixed diet, however, and it is not clear which dietary component is responsible either for the decrease in blood pressure or for any possible role in preventing coronary heart disease *(79)*.

Progression of coronary heart disease

Diet may indeed affect the progression of coronary atherosclerosis. In the Leiden study *(80)*, people at high risk of coronary atherosclerosis showed progressive narrowing of their coronary vessels when the ratio of total cholesterol to high-density lipoprotein (HDL) cholesterol in their blood was persistently high. Those who maintained a low ratio or who changed their ratio from high to low arrested the usual growth of the atherosclerotic lesion. The prognostic significance of HDL cholesterol was recognized some years ago by Miller & Miller *(81)* and has been observed in reanalyses of other surveys. One theory for this effect is that the concentration of HDL cholesterol reflects the rate at which cholesterol moves from the peripheral tissues to the liver for catabolism; the concentration of HDL cholesterol is low in people at high risk of coronary heart disease. Concentrations are low in obese people, and are reduced by physical inactivity and by smoking. Diet as such has a less obvious effect, although there are reports of an increase in concentrations of HDL cholesterol when intakes of saturated fatty acids fall and intakes of polyunsaturated fatty acids increase. Concentrations of HDL cholesterol usually rise with increased vitamin C intakes. In the Leiden study, a fall in the ratio of total cholesterol to HDL cholesterol was achieved mainly by altering the diet of the subjects to reduce the concentration of cholesterol in the very-low-density lipoproteins *(80)*.

The relationship between obesity and changes in total and in HDL cholesterol are illustrated in Fig. 31, which shows the results of a study of 7735 men aged 40–59 years in 24 towns in England, Scotland and Wales *(82)*. Increasing degrees of overweight were associated with increased levels of total serum cholesterol until the men reached a BMI of 28, after which the level stabilized. HDL cholesterol also declined progressively with increasing obesity.

Intervention studies
The idea that a diet rich in saturated fat leads to coronary heart disease and that the dietary effects are exacerbated by smoking and high blood pressure was based on associations arising from epidemiological, metabolic and experimental studies. The concept clearly needed further practical testing in the community before any preventive policy could be developed. Three kinds of intervention have been made over the last 15 years in Europe to assess the role of diet: selective action for people at high risk, advice for specified groups within the community without regard as to whether individuals are at high or low risk, and, finally, educational campaigns for the whole community.

High-risk strategy: the Oslo trial
An intervention study on men at high risk was conducted in Oslo *(83)*; 16 202 men aged 40–49 years were screened for coronary risk factors. Of these, 1232 men with high serum cholesterol levels (7.5–9.8 mmol/litre, or 290–380 mg/dl) were chosen for the study. They were randomly assigned to the intervention or control group. The intervention group received a total of 45 minutes' assessment, and advice on diet and smoking cessation when applicable. The dietary advice included a reduction in saturated fat, a slight increase in polyunsaturated fat intake, and a reduction in total energy intake from sugar, alcohol and fat in those with hypertriglyceridaemia. All were recommended to switch to high-fibre breads, to use skimmed milk

74

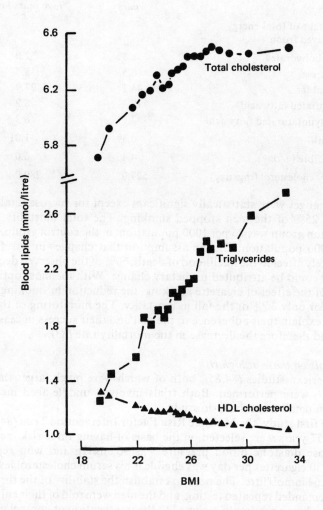

Fig. 31. The relationships between levels of blood lipids and BMI

Source: Thelle et al. *(82).*

and to reduce eggs to one per week. The wives of subjects in the intervention group were invited to a group discussion of methods of changing the diet.

Follow-up visits were made at six-month intervals with checks on body weight, blood pressure, blood lipids and electrocardiogram. A personal serum cholesterol curve was drawn for each man to display his response to the intervention.

Four years into the trial, the differences in diet included:

	Starting values	Values four years later
Percentage of total energy derived from:		
carbohydrates	38.8	52.0
sucrose	6.5	8.3
total fat	44.1	27.9
saturated fatty acid	18.3	8.2
polyunsaturated fatty acid	7.1	8.3
P:S ratio	0.39	1.01
Crude fibre (g/day)	4.4	6.0
Dietary cholesterol (mg/day)	527.0	289.0

All the changes were statistically significant except for sucrose intakes. In addition, 25% of the men stopped smoking. The total mortality in the intervention group was 26 per 1000 population; in the control group, it was 38 per 1000 population. On the assumption that changes in risk factors immediately affected the likelihood of death, 60% of the observed decline in mortality could be attributed to dietary change. With the most optimistic analysis of the effect of cigarette smoking, the reduction in smoking could account for only 26% of the fall in mortality. The monitoring of the men may well explain their adherence to the diet and their success in ceasing to smoke and therefore the decrease in the mortality rate (83).

Other trials on those at high risk
Two American studies (84,85), both of which were much larger than the Oslo trial, were performed. Both trials involved middle-aged men, but differed in detail from the Oslo study.

In the first study, the Multiple Risk Factor Intervention Trial (84), men aged 35–57 years were selected on the basis of having three risk factors; a man whose diastolic blood pressure was 90 mmHg and who reported smoking 30 cigarettes per day was eligible if his serum cholesterol level was at least 7.64 mmol/litre. The need to establish the stability of the three risk factors demanded repeated testing, and the men were told of their enhanced risk before being randomly assigned to the intervention or control groups. Men in the control group were referred back to their physician for management, provided with all the details on risk factors. When this group was followed up, therefore, it was not surprising that, instead of the expected death rate of 31 per 1000 population per year, the control group had a death rate of 19 per 1000, associated with reductions in serum cholesterol, smoking rates and blood pressure. The intervention group, receiving standardized advice, showed greater reductions in the risk factors. As expected, the death rate from coronary heart disease was lower (12 per 1000 population per year), but this was not significantly different from the control group. The trial was designed on the assumption that the control group would not change its diet, smoking habits and treatment of hypertension. The study did not therefore prove the value of intervention, even in a high-risk group, but most experts agree that the overall effects were consistent with the concept of benefit from changes in diet.

The second important trial was organized by the Lipid Research Clinics (85). It involved the use of colestyramine, which reduces total serum cholesterol. In this trial, 3806 men aged 35–59 years with hypercholes-terlaemia were given dietary advice with or without colestyramine. Because men who responded well initially to dietary advice alone were excluded from the trial, the subjects were men who were relatively resistant to dietary management. Colestyramine reduced the death rate from heart disease in these men, but not total mortality, compared with the group using only dietary advice. There was, however, a significant inverse relationship between the degree of reduction in cholesterol from continued dieting (with or without colestyramine) and the death rate from heart disease. While some interpret this study as relevant to community-based intervention studies, others feel it is important only in the clinical management of hyperlipid-aemic patients.

Community-based studies: WHO European trial
The European collaborative trial (86,87) included over 60 000 men in 80 factories in 4 European countries: Belgium, Italy, Poland and the United Kingdom. Men aged 40–59 years were invited to have a cardiovascular examination. The factories were then randomized, and the men in the intervention group were subjected to a general campaign aimed at changing their habits: altering the diet to lower serum cholesterol, stopping smoking, reducing weight, increasing daily exercise and controlling hypertension. Men found to have multiple risk factors received additional advice from physicians. Parts of the trial began in 1971 when there was little or no public awareness in some countries of the importance of diet, nonsmoking, exercise and weight maintenance.

The amount of advice given to the population groups varied. Limited advice was given to men working in British factories. In Belgium and Italy health education was much more extensive and there were substantial changes in the risk factors. Levels of serum cholesterol, blood pressure and cigarette smoking fell. Much less change was achieved in the United Kingdom, where the major effect was on smoking habits. In the Belgian group, the incidence of coronary heart disease fell by 24% in the inter-vention group and total mortality was 17% lower than in the control group. In the British factories death rates continued to rise. In the Polish factories, the incidence of coronary heart disease fell by 15.5% in the intervention group. After six years, the final report showed that, in the 80 factories, the total incidence of coronary heart disease fell by 10.2%, mortality from coronary heart disease fell by 6.9%, and total deaths declined by 5.3% as a result of the intervention. The decline in the measured risk factors seemed to account for 62% of the observed fall in the incidence of coronary heart disease.

Community-wide health education: the North Karelia Project
The North Karelia Project was the first attempt in Europe to see whether a community-wide programme of health education could alter dietary patterns, limit smoking, increase exercise and improve the monitoring and management of high blood pressure. It provided clear evidence that a public health programme could lead to substantial changes in behaviour patterns. For example, the type of milk consumed by the community (in which farming predominates) in this region of Finland changed significantly; the consumption of skimmed milk increased as that of full-fat milk declined. In association with these dietary changes, the severity of two risk factors, high serum cholesterol and high blood pressure, declined and a much greater proportion of the population became nonsmokers. The intervention was diverse and novel and permeated the whole area through a variety of educational programmes involving schoolchildren and adult clinics, education at work, and press, radio and television programmes. Not unnaturally, news of the programme spread, and the Finnish people as a whole became more conscious of the possibilities of preventive medicine. The adjoining region of Kuopio, originally designated as a reference area, was also affected. The reduction in risk factors was more pronounced in North Karelia than in the rest of the country and was associated with a greater decline in death rates from coronary heart disease. On this basis, a community-wide programme would appear to be an effective means of changing national dietary patterns. Such a programme can be accompanied by a decline in the incidence of coronary heart disease.

Sceptics argue that even the North Karelia Project did not provide sufficient evidence to warrant the claim that dietary changes reduced the incidence of coronary heart disease. Many factors were altered in North Karelia, so specific dietary changes cannot be identified as the cause of the improved health in the region. The original reference area, Kuopio, which borders on North Karelia, did not show a statistically different response, and only when the rest of the country was included could the statistical significance of the change in coronary heart disease in North Karelia be substantiated. North Karelia also had a very high mortality rate from cardiovascular diseases so any preventive measure might have been expected to have a greater effect on the problem than elsewhere *(8)*. Most experts, however, accept that the North Karelia Project established an effective precedent for changing a community's lifestyle. The Project did not provide absolute proof of the specific effect of dietary changes but set a standard of community intervention for others to follow *(88)*.

Factors changing national rates of coronary heart disease
A recent analysis of the causes of the decline in the mortality rate from ischaemic heart disease in some countries *(89)* has carefully evaluated the effects of smoking and the potential benefits of coronary bypass surgery, intensive resuscitation of patients before they enter the hospital, improved medical therapy for angina and hypertension, and changes in lifestyle that lead to a reduction in serum cholesterol levels. This analysis has been applied to changes observed in the United States. By a series of independent

78

statistical calculations that assessed the possible impact of dietary and other changes, it was determined that the factors considered seem to have accounted for 93.5% of the observed mortality. The relative importance of each factor is set out in Table 18. The table shows that a decline of only 0.17 mmol/litre in the average concentration of serum cholesterol accounts for 30% of the estimated fall in mortality between 1968 and 1976. The average decline in men was about 0.1 mmol/litre and that in women, 0.25 mmol/litre. These estimated changes were based on national samples in the Health Examination Survey, conducted from 1960 to 1962, and the Health and Nutrition Examination Survey, conducted from 1971 to 1974. In addition, despite an increase in exercise, American men and women actually increased their body weight during this period, so it is difficult to ascribe any reduction in mortality to a more appropriate body weight.

Table 18. Estimated effects of certain medical interventions
and changes in lifestyle on mortality
from ischaemic heart disease, United States, 1968–1976

	No. of lives saved	Percentage observed decline in mortality
Medical interventions		
Use of coronary care units	85 000	13.5
Resuscitation and care before the patient enters hospital	25 000	4.0
Coronary artery bypass surgery	23 000	3.5
Medical treatment of clinical ischaemic heart disease	61 000	10.0
Treatment of hypertension	55 000	8.5
Total	249 000	39.5
Changes in lifestyle		
Reduction in serum cholesterol levels	190 000	30.0
Reduction in cigarette smoking	150 000	24.0
Total	340 000	54.0
Not explained or due to errors in preceding estimates	41 000	6.5
Grand total	630 000	100.0

Source: Goldman & Cook *(89)*.

Proof before making policy?
People have long debated whether a government should base public health policies on experts' judgement of the cause of a major health problem. It is natural to demand more stringent proof that a dietary factor is linked to disease. Delivering such proof is difficult, and even more so if a disease is multifactorial. More recently some physicians involved in making public policy have argued that the value of a preventive programme to a defined population should be proved before it is applied to a whole nation.

Most experts now consider it unrealistic to demand proof that a specific dietary change causes a decline in the incidence of coronary heart disease in a community. Maintaining a logical argument for identifying a specific responsible factor would require a defined and well documented change in only one dietary feature, and no change in any other risk factor. The people involved in developing public health policy consider the combined results of the previously mentioned intervention trials as sufficient to justify public policy and nutrition education programmes that are designed to reduce saturated fatty acid intake in countries in which coronary heart disease is a substantial problem.

National campaigns for the prevention of coronary heart disease

Norway
The Norwegian Parliament adopted a nutrition policy in 1975. As part of this policy, a nutrition education campaign was started in 1982, with the broad objective of influencing health through a better diet. The link between coronary heart disease and diet has been a feature of information on nutrition in Norway since the 1960s. The National Nutrition Council, formed in 1946, was responsible for publicizing the campaign to organizations and the general public through the mass media and through advertising, posters, books and meetings with schools at national and local level *(90)*. The campaign advises people to change their diets, to reduce the total fat intake to 35% of the total energy intake, to increase the relative proportion of unsaturated to saturated fat, and to increase the consumption of starches (cereals and potatoes) and vegetables. Sugar should be limited to less than 10% and protein should provide 10–15% of total energy intake.

The campaign is aided by food subsidies to stimulate the consumption of grain, vegetables and low-fat milk. Transport subsidies are also available to stores in outlying districts to ensure a selection of healthy food. Since the campaign started in 1982, the consumption of vegetables, fruit and low-fat milk has increased, and that of whole milk and margarine has decreased. Fat intakes have decreased from 41% of the total energy intake in 1974 to 37% in 1985.

Sweden
In Sweden, the National Board of Health and Welfare, with the help of nutritionists, the media and the food industry, tried to alter dietary practices and increase exercise through a diet and exercise campaign lasting eight years. Industry responded by producing a variety of low-fat products, and

much new literature on health education was provided. The results of this campaign were difficult to evaluate because no national screening programme existed at the time. Nevertheless, the overall effect of the campaign seems to have been disappointing. There was no decline in serum cholesterol. The average body weight actually increased and there was a small rise in the rate of coronary heart disease (91). This failure has led to more rigorous demands for major changes in food composition, and in taxation and other national economic policies.

Other countries, such as Ireland (92), are now formulating national health campaigns, but none aims to test the hypothesis that diet is linked to heart disease. All are based on the assumption that these links (between saturated fatty acid intake, total serum cholesterol and coronary heart disease) are valid.

Cerebrovascular Disease

The principal risk factor for stroke is high blood pressure. Hypertension is therefore an important determinant. Age and sex are also important factors; they have already been considered in relation to coronary heart disease. Yet other factors may be involved in the pathogenesis of stroke, but little work on them has been undertaken.

Hypertension

The causes of hypertension may be many, but the factor most frequently cited is salt intake. The hypothesis was developed over 80 years ago, and it has been recognized for decades that a salt-poor diet can be useful in the treatment of hypertension. This fact, however, does not necessarily mean that salt causes the condition. The role of salt in hypertension remains somewhat controversial; individual investigators suggest that the link is too tentative to allow public policy to be based on it (93). The WHO Expert Committee on Prevention of Coronary Heart Disease (94) felt sufficiently confident of the link, however, to advocate a reduction in the consumption of salt. This was confirmed by the WHO Scientific Group on Primary Prevention of Essential Hypertension (12).

Populations that do not show a rise in blood pressure with age have diets characterized by a low salt intake. No population with a low salt intake and a marked prevalence of hypertension has been discovered; nor has a population with a high salt intake been found to lack a major problem with hypertension in the community. Nevertheless, the populations that enjoy normal levels of blood pressure throughout life characteristically have a higher potassium intake, lower body weight and greater physical activity, as well as many other differences from conditions seen in Europe.

Gleiberman (95) highlighted the possible role of salt in the development of high blood pressure by relating estimates of salt consumption or measurements of 24-hour urinary sodium excretion to the average blood pressure of groups throughout the world. These estimates were very crude but they were backed by other research. A series of studies shows that, as people move from a low-salt diet in such areas as East Africa or the Pacific islands, and acquire a different pattern of life with an increase in sodium intake, their blood pressure begins to rise. Showing a correlation between salt intake and blood pressure within a population, however, has been much more difficult. This has often been ascribed to the need for careful, repeated measurements of blood pressure (to take account of its variability), and of 24-hour urine output (to ensure that the variation in salt intake in a particular person is adequately monitored). Recent studies have fulfilled these exacting criteria, but have still failed to show a clear correlation. This failure may reflect the importance of genetic susceptibility to salt. The findings of these studies do not disprove the proposition that dietary salt leads to hypertension in susceptible individuals.

Other factors are recognized as being involved in the development of hypertension: obesity and alcohol consumption. Recently, McCarron (96) has suggested that calcium intake is particularly important for minimizing the development of hypertension. The importance of a high ratio of potassium to sodium in the diet has also been emphasized (97,98). Another study suggests that a higher potassium intake is beneficial (99). Questions have also been raised as to whether the chloride or the sodium in salt is of greater etiological significance, and controlled feeding trials in individuals and in families have suggested that a high intake of saturated fat may be conducive to an increase in blood pressure (100). Puska et al. (101) and Iacono et al. (102) have found similar results. These additional factors may amplify or modify the process whereby salt induces hypertension. Until scientists discover whether and how they do so, the discussion must remain speculative.

Intervention studies provide some evidence of the importance of salt in the management of hypertension; unfortunately, the evidence tends to be conflicting (103). A reduction in blood pressure of 3–8 mmHg has been observed in several open and double-blind trials (104–108). However, interpreting these results is difficult. Most of the studies have been of short duration and the criteria for estimating salt intake have differed greatly. The double-blind study reported by MacGregor et al. (104) and the one-year open trial of Beard et al. (109) strongly suggest that salt restriction is indeed of benefit in the treatment of hypertension. It is therefore surprising that several other studies (101,110–112) have observed no change in the blood pressure of hypertensive, borderline hypertensive or normotensive subjects despite well documented reductions in salt intake, urinary salt excretion or both.

Prospective and intervention studies have included an analysis of the effects of salt on the blood pressure of children. When babies were provided with either a low-sodium diet or normal-sodium diet for the first six months of life, the blood pressure of the normal-sodium group was 2 mmHg higher than that of the low-sodium group, and there were statistically significant differences in the rate of increase in blood pressure from birth. In adults, Joossens & Geboers (113) consider that the reduction in salt intake in northern Belgium has led to a fall in average blood pressure. The dietary changes were not confined to salt, however, so the change in salt intake has not been established as the major factor. Similar doubts have been cast on the North Karelia Project in Finland, which also involved many changes. Nevertheless, with a reduction in salt intake and a change in the amount and type of fat eaten, the number of hypertensives and the mean blood pressure of this community have dropped appreciably.

Diabetes

The differences between the two types of diabetes mellitus have already been noted. The importance of viral infections in precipitating insulin-dependent diabetes in genetically susceptible people has also been mentioned; few studies imply any involvement of dietary factors. In Iceland, however, the ingestion of nitrosamines (derived from cured mutton and consumed by both men and women) when women conceive has been suggested to lead to genetic changes in the offspring that make them susceptible to diabetes in later years *(114)*. Some animal experiments support this unusual idea, but no further work seems to have been undertaken.

Poor nutrition has always been considered a major risk factor for the majority of diabetics with non-insulin-dependent diabetes mellitus. Obesity has long been accepted as a major precipitating factor; the risk is related to both the duration and the degree of obesity. According to a WHO study group, obesity induces resistance to the action of insulin by a variety of mechanisms, including reductions in the number of insulin receptors and, more often, postreceptor changes *(13)*. The precise causes of this resistance are unknown, but may include an increased storage of fat, increased energy intake, the composition of the diet (especially high fat intake), and physical inactivity. No sound evidence associates diabetes with a high intake of any of the major nutrients, such as sucrose. Resistance to insulin is recognized to be reduced by restricting the diet, which leads to weight loss. Physical training and controlling blood sugar levels with insulin or with sulfonylureas are also effective. If remedial measures are not adopted, the beta cells in the pancreas of a genetically predisposed person may not be able to meet the chronic challenge of insulin resistance. Diabetes may then result.

High and low rates of diabetes have been linked to a number of social factors, including occupation, marital status, religion, economic status and the level of education. Although diabetes is frequently discovered during pregnancy, most evidence suggests that parity is not a risk factor for the condition.

Obesity

There are no satisfactory explanations for the marked differences in the prevalence of obesity in different parts of Europe. Studies sponsored by FAO[a] suggest that the weight-for-height of men, women and children relates to the proportion of energy derived from dietary fat, irrespective of the other social factors that are known to be linked to the prevalence rate of obesity.

---

[a] François, P. (personal communication).

Obesity has many causes. Dietary variety, for example, tends to increase food intake. A high energy density from an excess of dietary sugar, as well as dietary fat, is generally considered to be conducive to the development of obesity. Physical inactivity is also widely recognized as important, and these environmental factors interact with people's genetic predisposition. Of course, the interaction of dietary and other environmental factors with genetic propensity can be noted in almost all of the conditions considered in this publication.

Cancer

Many environmental factors, including diet, have now been linked to the development of cancer. The difficulty with making any claims about the links between diet and cancer is that so little is known about the subject. The incidence of various types of cancer, as already demonstrated, varies among countries. Environmental factors are very important, but identifying them and then assessing their quantitative significance is extremely difficult. Doll & Peto *(115)* have attempted to do this on a statistical basis. They consider that perhaps 35% of all types of cancer may eventually be linked to dietary factors, but their acceptable estimates range from 10% to 70%. In contrast, they blame tobacco for 30% of cancer, with a range of acceptable estimates from 25% to 40%. Further, Doll & Peto consider that alcohol may account for 3% of cancers and food additives for perhaps only 1%. The additional problems of food contamination and industrial pollution may only account for a further 1%. Brzeziński[a] has also summarized the many occupational causes of cancer, but dietary factors do not in general seem either to amplify or to limit these.

Breast cancer

The importance of environmental factors in breast cancer is clear, because its incidence changes in migrants as they move from low-risk to high-risk countries and change their diet. Dietary fat has been widely cited as important in the development of breast cancer. This work is, however, based predominantly on epidemiological research and animal experiments. Fig. 32 shows the high correlation between estimated saturated fat intake and age-adjusted death rates for breast cancer in 23 European countries. This does not necessarily mean, however, that saturated fatty acids play an important role in the development of breast cancer; other associated dietary factors may prove to be important.

Case-control studies also link an increased risk of breast cancer with excessive fat intake, the epidemiological link being more apparent after the menopause than before it *(18)*. Animal experiments are based primarily on studies in which breast cancer is induced by specific carcinogens *(116)*; dietary fat is then found to promote the development of mammary tumours. In

---

[a] **Brzeziński, Z.J.** *Regional targets in support of the regional strategy for health for all: epidemiological background.* Copenhagen, WHO Regional Office for Europe, 1984 (unpublished document EUR/RC34/Conf.Doc./5).

Fig. 32. Saturated fat in the diet and breast cancer mortality rates
per 100 000 population, females, 30–64 years,
in 23 countries, 1975–1979

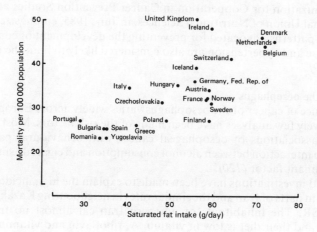

Note.   Saturated fat intake calculated from *Food balance sheets 1979–81 average (3)*.

experiments, diets rich in polyunsaturated fats promote tumours more
effectively than those rich in saturated fats. The mechanisms suggested for
these changes are many. They include changes in the lipid content of the cell
membrane, the synthesis of prostaglandins, the immune system, gut flora,
bile acid metabolism, and the recycling of steroidal metabolites.

It is also suggested that endocrine links could be mediated through a
fat-induced change in the secretion of prolactin and estrogen. Prolactin is
considered to induce breast cancer and estrogen to protect women from it.
In human studies *(18)*, increases in peak prolactin concentration during the
early morning hours are particularly common in women with diets high in
fat; this greater stimulus may promote the development of breast cancer in
susceptible people. Vegetarians have a lower prolactin level and are recognized to have a lower breast cancer rate. Differences in prolactin profile have
also been found in different cultures, but it is by no means clear that these
differences in vegetarians and in different cultures depend solely on differences in fat intake.

This circumstantial evidence led the Committee on Diet, Nutrition, and
Cancer in the United States to suggest that the link between dietary fat and
breast cancer incidence should be taken seriously *(117)*. Indeed, on the basis
of the geographical association and the experimental evidence, the Committee recommended a reduction in the fat content of the diet of Americans.
It seems that only in Sweden has an officially appointed group of scientists
made a similar analysis of risk *(118)*. The Swedish group concluded that diet
has a substantial effect in determining total cancer incidence, but could not
give precise figures on this. Cautious conclusions could be drawn about

the significant dietary components. Lowering fat intake was considered the most urgent dietary recommendation, accompanied by an increase in the consumption of cereals, fruit and vegetables. A joint meeting of the European Organization for Cooperation in Cancer Prevention Studies and the International Union of Nutritional Sciences, in June 1985, emphasized that the dietary patterns advocated for preventing the development of coronary heart disease and hypertension are also considered likely to limit the risk of cancer *(119)*.

Cancer of the oesophagus
The incidence of cancer of the oesophagus varies widely across Europe, but comparatively few analyses have been made of the risk factors. Most of the statistical associations of oesophageal cancer with behavioural patterns point to the interaction between alcohol consumption and cigarette smoking as the dominant factor *(120)*.

Detailed investigations have been made to explain the high incidence of this cancer in parts of Iran and the similar rates in neighbouring Kazakhstan, in the USSR. The inhabitants of northern Iran eat almost no fruit or vegetables and their diet is low in vitamin A, riboflavin and vitamin C, as well as in animal protein. Cook-Mozaffari *(15)* discovered that people in the high incidence area characteristically had very high intakes of opium, which could be assessed only by measuring metabolic products in urine. Over half of the adult men and women aged over 35 years were shown to have used opium in the previous 24 hours; these people seem to ingest the residue scraped from the inside of opium pipes. Local carcinogenic effects may thus be more important than any dietary component, but mild vitamin deficiencies may accentuate the effects of the carcinogen. No significantly high concentrations of nitrosamines, aflatoxins or polycyclic hydrocarbons were found in these areas. The principal causes of oesophageal cancer may differ from country to country.

Rates of oesophageal cancer are high in some regions of France *(15)*, but there is no clear association with alcohol consumption. High alcohol intakes do coincide with high death rates from oesophageal cancer in Normandy and Brittany, but not in the Ardennes and the French Alps. The nature of local drinks may be important, but no definitive findings have yet been reported.

Cancer of the stomach
Many hypotheses of dietary factors in cancer of the stomach have been put forward, and Fig. 33 summarizes some of the suggested factors that may promote or inhibit the development of cancer of the stomach. This is a theoretical scheme which has yet to be tested fully. Nitrate intake is readily converted to nitrite by bacterial action and recycles via the saliva. Gastric acid inhibits the growth of bacteria within the stomach and thereby limits the potential for nitrosamine formation. Nitrosamine induction may be promoted by the bacterial proliferation in the stomach of a hypochlorhydric person. Joossens *(121)* has suggested that salt could also be linked with stomach cancer because it induces gastric atrophy. Although the incidence rate of stomach cancer in Japan is remarkably high, detailed metabolic

86

Fig. 33. Diet and cancer of the stomach

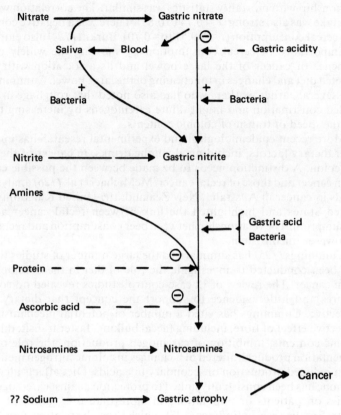

Dietary factor

studies have not been made to assess the dietary factors that might lead to metaplasia of the gastric mucosa. Vitamin C intakes may protect people from gastric cancer by limiting the production of nitrite from nitrate, but the relative importance of these dietary factors remains unclear. A case-control study in Greece *(122)* found, as have other studies, lower consumption of fruit, vegetables and cereals in patients with cancer and a greater consumption of pasta, beans and nuts. These features are consistent with the international variations in incidence rates. The rapid change and progressive decline in the incidence and death rates for stomach cancer throughout the world is noteworthy.

Cancer of the large bowel

Armstrong & Doll *(123)*, in their analysis of the environmental factors in cancer incidence in different countries, based the statistical correlations with diet on FAO food balance sheets as an indirect estimate of food consumption. They found a correlation in a number of countries between meat consumption and colon cancer ($r = 0.85$ in men and $r = 0.89$ in women). The relationship with mortality statistics was similar. The correlation with total fat intake was also strong ($r = 0.74$ to 0.85). There was a negative correlation with cereal consumption ($r = -0.51$ to -0.70). Burkitt (124) also emphasized the importance of cereal consumption by showing the widely differing incidence of cancer of the large bowel and its association with a fibre-depleted diet and changes in functioning of the large bowel. Cummings (125) cites several earlier workers who had also noted that roughage in the diet limited constipation and might dilute carcinogens by increasing the bulk and the speed of transit of colonic contents.

More recent epidemiological and experimental research has implicated other dietary factors, including alcoholic drinks, in cancer of the rectum and colon. A distinction needs to be made between the possible causes of colon cancer and those of rectal cancer. McMichael et al. (126) analysed time trends in cancer in Australia, New Zealand, the United Kingdom and the United States and highlighted the link between rectal cancer and beer consumption. The relationship between beer consumption and rectal cancer is, however, inconsistent.

Cummings (125) has summarized the large number of studies that have now been conducted to investigate the role of diet in the development of colon cancer. The review of 12 case-control studies revealed no consistent features and little evidence to support the concept that dietary fibre is protective. Cummings has cited a number of potential mechanisms for a protective effect of fibre, including faecal bulking, faster transit, dilution of colonic contents, inhibition of carcinogen production, the role of fibre's fermentation products, altered pH, changes in colonic nitrogen metabolism, and a reduced production of secondary bile acids. Diet affects all of these, but none has been consistently linked to protection against carcinogenesis in studies on patients or populations in more than one continent. Fig. 34 illustrates some recent findings (127), which show the relationships between faecal bile acid concentration, stool weight and the incidence of colon cancer in two Danish and two Finnish populations (one rural and one in the capital of each country) and in New Yorkers. New analyses, using modern techniques for measuring dietary fibre, suggest an inverse relationship between fibre intake and colon cancer incidence. If this relationship is significant, then the high intake of rye bread in the Finns in rural Kuopio may protect them from cancer of the colon, despite their high fat intake. It does not, however, seem to protect them against coronary heart disease. Cummings (125) points out that all studies do not show a protective effect of fibre and high faecal bulk. For example, the Maoris in New Zealand have a high colon cancer rate but a fibre intake and stool weight similar to those of the white New Zealanders, who have a lower rate of colon cancer. The causes of this cancer may, of course, differ from one country to another.

Dietary fat promotes the development of colon cancer in experimental animals, but other factors may be involved. Mutagens have been found in barbecued meat, and vitamins A and E and dietary calcium have all been

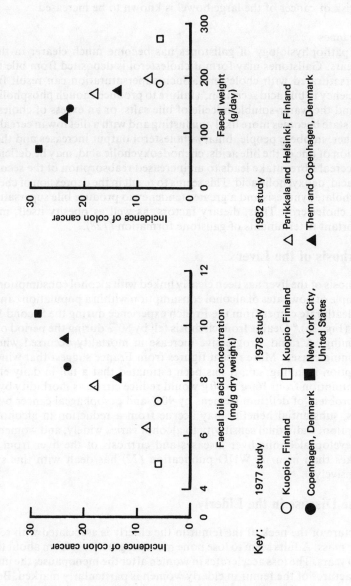

Fig. 34. The relationship between faecal bile acid concentration and faecal weight and the incidence of colon cancer in three studies, made in 1977, 1978 and 1982

1977 study

Key:
○ Kuopio, Finland
● Copenhagen, Denmark

1978 study
□ Kuopio Finland
■ New York City, United States

1982 study
△ Parikkala and Helsinki, Finland
▲ Them and Copenhagen, Denmark

Source: Muir & James (*127*).

proposed as possibly protective. Research continues on the dietary and metabolic factors linked to the development of colon cancer, but studies are not easy to make; a large number of people must be studied in detail to pick up the individuals who later develop cancer of the colon. Dietary trials are therefore now mainly confined to individuals with polyposis coli, in which the risk of cancer of the large bowel is known to be increased.

Gallstones
The pathophysiology of gallstones has become much clearer in the last 30 years. Gallstones may form if cholesterol is deposited from bile that is supersaturated with cholesterol. Such supersaturation can result from a deficiency in bile acid secretion, a failure to produce enough phospholipid to expand the water-soluble micelle of bile salts, or an excess of cholesterol. This state becomes more likely on fasting and with a diet low in cereal fibre. Further, in obese people, biliary cholesterol output increases and the production of one of the bile acids, chenodeoxycholic acid, may be deficient. A low cereal fibre intake leads to an increased reabsorption of the secondary bile acid, deoxycholic acid. This seems to result in the depression of chenodeoxycholate synthesis and a greater tendency to produce bile supersaturated with cholesterol. Thus, dietary factors, as well as obesity itself, may be important determinants of gallstone formation *(128)*.

Cirrhosis of the Liver

Cirrhosis of the liver has been clearly linked with alcohol consumption. One example of how rates of alcohol consumption within a population can affect the death rate comes from the French experience during the Second World War (Fig. 35).[a] Deaths from cirrhosis fell by 80% during the period of wine rationing. A rapid, progressive increase in mortality occurred when the rationing ceased. More recent figures from France suggest that wine consumption is falling, and it has been estimated that a fall in daily ethanol consumption from 160 g to 80 g would reduce cirrhosis morbidity by 58%, the problem of delirium tremens by 90% and oesophageal cancer by 28%. Thus, substantial benefits may accrue from a reduction in alcohol consumption. Individual sensitivity to alcohol varies widely, and women seem to develop alcoholic liver diseases and cirrhosis of the liver from lower intakes than men. A WHO publication *(22)* has dealt with this subject extensively.

Bone Disease in the Elderly

Fracture of the neck of the femur in the elderly is associated with reduced bone mass. Adults seem to lose bone mass progressively from about the age of 30 years. The loss accelerates in women after the menopause; the increase in fractures of the femur in elderly women is particularly marked. Below a critical level of bone mass, there is an increased likelihood of "spontaneous"

---

[a] Nguyen, J.-F. (personal communication).

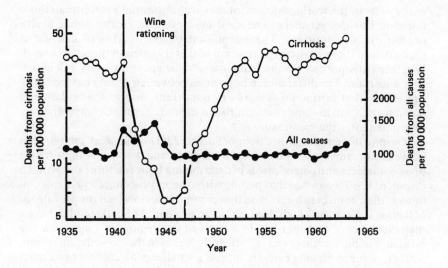

Fig. 35. General mortality, and mortality from cirrhosis of the liver, Paris, 1935–1963

Source: Nguyen, J.-F. (personal communication).

fractures of the hip and vertebrae. The factors determining the loss of bone mass are therefore likely to be important if fractures are to be prevented. The accumulation of a substantial bone mass in childhood and early adult life should prevent the total bone mass from falling to the critical level later in life. Environmental factors, including diet, could affect both the accumulation and loss of bone mass.

Physical activity and a good supply of dietary calcium have both been cited as important throughout life. The calcium intake needed to maintain metabolic balance is higher in women than in men and increases with age in both sexes, particularly after the menopause in women. The proposal that older people need more calcium is inferred from the observed decline in the efficiency of calcium absorption. Thus, the mean requirement for pre-menopausal women aged 35–50 years has been estimated to be about 1000 mg per day (implying a recommended allowance of about 1400 mg per day) *(129)*. The estimated requirement increases by about 50% in post-menopausal women. These requirements are substantially greater than recommended intakes (500 mg per day in the United Kingdom, for example) and the observed dietary supply in many European countries. The higher values are based not on balance studies, which assess the minimum intake compatible with calcium balance, but on a series of dietary studies and therapeutic trials geared to limiting the loss of bone mass. Large doses of calcium thus seem to be required to limit the loss of bone in both normal and osteoporotic people *(130)* and to reduce the incidence of vertebral fractures. This does not necessarily mean, however, that an intake below that level is the primary factor leading to osteoporosis. It must be remembered that, in many parts of the world, calcium intakes are substantially lower than those found in Europe, yet there is no clear evidence of a greater public health problem of osteoporosis. The adaptation to low intakes of calcium is gradual, and thereby alters the fraction of dietary calcium that is absorbed. Whether osteoporosis results from a true deficiency of dietary calcium is very uncertain. The difference in bone mass between the sexes has led to the suggestion that hormonal factors are important, and to the widespread recommendation in some communities to use estrogen replacement therapy on women after the menopause.

Despite this emphasis on calcium, Parfitt *(129)* notes a weak relationship between calcium intake and cortical bone mass, and the relative importance of osteomalacia and osteoporosis in determining bone fracture rates is much disputed. It is recognized that people with osteoporosis have lower calcium intakes than control subjects, and that communities in which the prevalence of lactase deficiency is high, leading to the avoidance of milk, tend to have a high incidence of osteoporosis. In a study of two regions in Yugoslavia the incidence of hip fractures was significantly higher in the low-calcium region; further, reduced lifelong calcium intake, a smaller peak cortical bone mass in adults and the prevalence of osteoporosis seemed to be related *(131)*.

Studies in the United Kingdom have shown that elderly patients with reduced bone mass may also have subclinical vitamin D deficiency, and thus an increased risk of hip fracture. Parfitt et al. *(132)* consider that the risk is mediated not by osteomalacia but by the accelerated loss of cortical bone induced by secondary hyperparathyroidism as the body attempts to respond to the low intake of dietary calcium. The correction of vitamin D depletion in the elderly has not yet been formally tested, however, to see whether it prevents fractures of the femur. A reduced phosphate intake has also been linked to osteoporosis. Dietary protein has also been cited as increasing calcium loss, since a higher protein intake is accompanied by a higher intake of sulfur-containing amino acids. When metabolized, these act as an acid load. An increase in sodium intake also seems to enhance calcium output. It has been suggested, however, that these experimental studies may not be relevant to normal diets that contain a substantial number of buffering factors *(133)*. The intake of fluoride has also been suggested as a protective factor *(134)* and fluoride has been successfully included in the drug therapy of osteoporosis *(135)*. Recent studies also suggest that people with osteoporosis may be deficient in vitamin K, but this preliminary finding has been neither substantiated nor tested in epidemiological or therapeutic trials.

The slower loss of cortical bone mass in lacto/ovo/vegetarians may reflect a high intake of calcium from milk, a lower intake of sulfur-containing amino acids because of meat avoidance, or a high intake of fibre, with its potential for buffering. It is known that Eskimos lose cortical bone rapidly with age, in association with their high meat consumption, but a number of other explanations may also be important. Vitamin C deficiency has been linked to a reduced bone mass in children with scurvy, but it is not clear whether this is important in the elderly.

Parfitt et al. *(132)* have concluded that, while very low or very high intakes of many nutrients are harmful to bone, the variation in the intake of nutrients (except calcium) seen in most European populations is unlikely to have a major effect. A recent Consultation organized by the WHO Regional Office for Europe[a] suggested that the prevention of osteoporosis will depend on a health policy that emphasizes the factors related to modern lifestyles, such as smoking, physical inactivity, and a diet low in calcium and/or too high in protein. All these factors affect the development of osteoporosis. The WHO Consultation did not, however, consider that the evidence warranted a recommendation to increase the allowance of calcium above the 600 mg per day usually proposed by expert groups in northern European countries. Exposing the skin to sunlight, to maintain vitamin D stores throughout the year, was also considered important but this seasonal storage of vitamin D is less readily achieved in northern Europe. Vitamin D status depends mainly on exposing the skin to ultraviolet light of a specific wavelength, which is very limited in northern latitudes during the winter months. Vitamin D deficiency is sufficiently common among the elderly to warrant advising them to expose themselves to reasonable amounts of sun when feasible. This approach is preferable to the widespread use of oral supplements of vitamin D; if used unwisely, these can lead to vitamin D toxicity.

Oral Disease

A vast amount of evidence from a wide range of sources (observational and interventional studies on human populations, animal studies, plaque pH and *in vitro* experiments) incriminates sugar in the development of dental caries *(136–138)*. Virtually all dental researchers are agreed on the importance of this relationship, which was also endorsed by a joint FAO/WHO report *(139)*. The process of demineralization of hydroxyapatite in tooth enamel depends on the production of acid. This acid is generated within the dental plaque by bacterial fermentation of carbohydrates. There is also evidence that sucrose is particularly conducive to the implantation and growth of the bacteria responsible for producing the plaque. Once plaque is formed, oral bacteria rapidly metabolize any simple sugar (such as sucrose, glucose or fructose) to acids *(136)*. The generation of acids reduces the pH to less than 5.5; at this point demineralization of the tooth begins. Eating sucrose on more than three occasions a day reduces the pH of the plaque to below 5.5 for more than three hours a day. Sugar alcohols, such as sorbitol, mannitol and xylitol, and intense sweeteners are usually classified as noncariogenic.

A large number of factors can influence the development of dental caries. These include the frequency of simple sugar intake, the degree of

---

[a] **Davies, L.S. & Holdsworth, M.D.** *Prevention of osteoporosis — a nutrition/public health concern.* Copenhagen, WHO Regional Office for Europe, 1984 (unpublished document ICP/NUT 102/m01).

stimulation of salivary flow, the composition of saliva, the stickiness of the food being ingested, the chemical structure of the enamel, the degree of fluoridation of water, hereditary factors, and the amount of care taken with oral hygiene. It is therefore not surprising that an epidemiological relationship between total sucrose intakes and the prevalence of dental caries, such as that shown in Fig. 21, shows inconsistent results. Similar analyses (140) show a poor relationship, and population studies on groups in the United States (141) have emphasized that the form of sugar and frequency of consumption are more important than the total amount consumed. In the United Kingdom, the Dental Strategy Review Group of the Department of Health and Social Security also advocates a specific reduction in sugar intake between meals.

Given this complexity, how can quantitative guidelines appropriate for a whole population be developed? This problem applies to many of the links currently being made between inappropriate intakes of nutrients and the slow development of disease. Epidemiological data, some of it cross-sectional, must be used, and supplemented when possible with longitudinal studies and intervention trials. Many analyses and trials have been conducted (141–145); as a result, different workers have proposed that the average intake of sugar should fall to below 30 g per person per day (139,143) or 50 g per person per day (28). Sheiham (136) proposes that, in countries in which fluoride is added to toothpastes, there is less need to endorse very restricted intakes of sugar; he suggests 40 g as an average daily per capita intake for a community. Fig. 36 shows the relationship between the annual sugar consumption and the incidence of dental caries in Japanese schoolchildren (146). This analysis was conduced on 7894 boys and girls when there was a low intake of sugar; Japanese sugar intakes appear to have risen appreciably since then. Sognnaes (147) reviewed 27 studies from 11 European countries covering 750 000 children. Reductions in the prevalence and severity of caries were observed in all studies in which the period of observation covered the years of the Second World War, when sugar intakes fell. Most studies on young children aged up to five years have also shown significant correlations between caries and exposure to sugar. In older children, however, there was a poorer correlation.

The British Association for the Study of Community Dentistry (148) reviewed the human clinical studies on the link between sugar and dental caries and noted that the large Vipeholm study (149) had clearly shown that consumption of sugar, even at high levels, was associated with only a small increase in caries if sugar was taken up to four times a day at mealtimes only. In contrast, the consumption of sugar both between meals and at meals was associated with a marked increase in caries. The Turku study (150) demonstrated that xylitol, but not fructose, was less cariogenic than sucrose. When chewing-gum containing xylitol rather than sucrose was provided, pre-cavitation lesions in the teeth healed during the one-year test period. This indicated that chewing a gum that did not produce acid but provoked a strong salivary response may aid the remineralization of enamel. A two-year British study tested the effect on the development of caries of supplementing children's diet with additional sugar (151). The study suggested that, even

Fig. 36. Annual incidence of caries in first molars
in Japanese schoolchildren and the
annual sugar consumption in Japan, 1941–1958

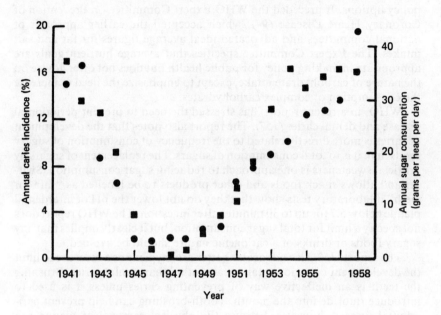

Source: Rugg-Gunn *(146).*

when the sugar intake was doubled, there was no clear increase in caries
incidence over a period of up to two years. The sugar, however, was only
given at mealtimes. This supports the findings of the Vipeholm study, that
restricting sugar to mealtimes does not lead to a marked increase in caries.
Exposing teeth to sucrose solutions nine times a day, however, leads to an
increase in carious lesions *(152,153).*

Although new methods are being developed to measure the relative
cariogenicity of different foods *(152,154),* there is no prospect of early
success. Health educators need to continue their efforts to increase the use of
fluoride, to improve oral hygiene, and to limit the consumption of sweets,
soft drinks, and snacks that contain simple sugars. The reasons for the
proposal, by a Swedish group *(155)* dealing with nutritional guidelines, of
10% for the energy derived from sugar was based on other nutritional
considerations. The common Nordic nutrient recommendations of 1980
(156) also suggest a 10% figure for sugar intakes, a value similar to that

95

proposed by the Obesity Working Party (56) of the Royal College of Physicians in the United Kingdom. The 1980 FAO/WHO report on carbohydrates makes no mention of nutrient goals or dietary guidelines (139). The report is a brief scientific review of carbohydrates rather than an analysis of policy options. It preceded the WHO Expert Committee on Prevention of Coronary Heart Disease (94), which accepted the earlier approach of national committees and advocated ideal average figures for fat and salt intakes. The Expert Committee specifies that average nutrient goals are appropriate in making policy for public health but does not offer advice on the nature of carbohydrate intake, except to emphasize the need to increase the consumption of complex carbohydrates.

WHO, in a recent report, has stressed the need to prevent periodontal disease and dental caries (157). The report also notes that the development of caries is more directly related to the frequency of consumption of sugary foods than it is to total consumption of sugars. The replacement of sugars by artificial sweeteners is one approach to reducing sugar consumption. Switzerland allows snack foods and other products to be labelled as "safe for teeth" if laboratory tests show that they do not lower the pH of interdental plaque below 5.7 for up to 30 minutes after ingestion. The WHO report does not specify a limit for total sugar consumption, but it clearly implies that any sugary foods or drinks of a cariogenic nature should be avoided.

The report (157) also advocates better oral hygiene as a measure to limit the development of periodontal disease rather than dental caries. Brushing the teeth is an ineffective way of preventing caries unless it is used to introduce fluoride into the mouth. Tooth-brushing can help prevent periodontal disease, however, because the physical removal of plaque can reduce the development and progression of the disease.

Apart from dietary measures, the use of fluoride (in water, tablets, toothpaste, salt or mouth rinses) can play an important part in preventing dental caries. An extensive WHO report (158) deals with the optimum intake of fluoride, suggesting that drinking-water should contain 0.7–1.2 mg fluoride per litre, depending on climatic conditions.

WHO and the International Dental Federation have developed global goals for achieving oral health objectives for the year 2000 (159). These five goals relate to five specific age groups: children of 5–6 years, 12 years and 18 years and adults aged 35–44 and over 65. The goal for the last group, for example, is to reduce the proportion of the elderly population found to be edentulous to 75% of the 1981 figure. This illustrates the importance of a pragmatic approach to the development of targets or goals.

Nutritional Anaemia

Iron deficiency is the principal nutritional cause of anaemia, followed by folic acid deficiency. In some European countries, haemolytic anaemia may develop in genetically susceptible people after they eat the broad bean, *Vicia fava*. This last form of anaemia is particularly common in the Mediterranean area, where the condition is known as favism. The differences in prevalence of iron deficiency in Europe are mostly dietary in origin. The prevalence of intestinal parasitism in different nations is unknown but is considered unlikely to be a major factor in European countries, as distinct from developing countries. Intestinal parasitism increases dietary iron requirements. Other factors, such as the use of hormonal contraceptives in women, tend to reduce iron requirements. The Pill reduces menstrual losses by about 50%, and in one Finnish study (37) the haemoglobin level was 1.9 g/litre higher in the 11% of the menstruating women who used the Pill; this difference was statistically significant. Intrauterine devices, however, may increase menstrual loss by about 100%.

In the Heidelberg study (39), a larger proportion of the women (38%) was taking the Pill when tested, but these women did not differ from others in haematocrit readings or haemoglobin levels. Differences in the proportion of pregnant women or in the use of iron supplements may also explain regional differences in the prevalence of anaemia.

In men and in postmenopausal women in Europe, anaemia may not be nutritional in origin; it may develop as a secondary manifestation of an infection and is particularly evident in the elderly. This secondary anaemia is accompanied by a low level of plasma iron and a low rather than a high concentration of plasma transferrin. Where true iron-deficiency anaemia occurs in European populations, it is usually possible to find a source of intestinal bleeding, such as an ulcer, a tumour or diverticulitis of the colon.

Dietary intake of iron

Haem iron, derived from haemoglobin and myoglobin, is more easily absorbed than the nonhaem iron derived from cereals, fruits and vegetables. The second form normally accounts for 85–90% of dietary iron and its absorption is markedly influenced by other dietary factors. Haem iron is well absorbed and relatively unaffected by the inhibitory effects of phytate, phosphate, tannins and other dietary components that can determine a sevenfold range in the amount of iron absorbed (160). Meat, as well as supplying haem iron, enhances the absorption of nonhaem iron, but the most important promoter of iron uptake is vitamin C. Adding vitamin C to a meal markedly increases the amount of inorganic iron absorbed, but the fraction absorbed also reflects the state of iron stores in the body. As tissue iron is depleted, adaptive changes occur that increase the proportion of iron extracted from food by the intestine.

Different intakes of iron and of foods known to affect the bioavailability of iron are relevant to the prevalence rates of anaemia in different countries, despite the problems of comparing such rates. In Sweden, Norway and Finland, for example, just as meat intake is lower than in many other European countries, so is the intake of dietary haem iron. Data on the average intake of foods and drinks known to inhibit iron absorption because of their phytate and tannin content (such as bran, certain vegetables, tea and coffee) would also be valuable if information were available.

The changes in food patterns in European countries over the last 30 years have already been noted. Table 19 provides further evidence that may relate to the changing availability of iron (38,39,161–163). Meat intake increased in Sweden until recently, when a decline began. Iron from cereals has also

Table 19. Daily dietary iron intake from different sources of food

| Sources of iron | Consumption data for all Sweden[a] | | | | | | | | Women in: | | | | | | | |
| | 1960 | | 1970 | 1980[b] | 1980[b] | 1982 | 1984 | | Sweden 1963[c] | | Fed. Rep. of Germany 1978–1979[d] | | France 1985[e] | | Denmark 1985[f] | |
	mg	%	mg	mg	mg	mg	mg	%	mg	%	mg	%	mg	%	mg	%
Meat	3.0	23.4	3.3	3.7	3.2	3.2	3.0	15	2.8	24.4	4.0	30.1	3.2	29.5	2.2	17
Fish	0.4	3.1	0.4	0.4	0.4	0.4	0.4	2	}	}	}	}	}	}	0.1	1
Eggs	0.7	5.5	0.7	0.7	0.6	0.6	0.6	3	0.6	5.2			0.8	7.3	0.5	4
Vegetables, fruit and roots	3.3	25.8	3.5	3.4	4.0	3.8	3.8	19	2.4	20.9	1.8	13.5	3.5	31.8	2.1	16
Cereals	4.5	35.2	7.2	9.1	9.7	10.0	10.0	51	3.7	32.1	3.4	25.6	1.9	17.8	6.6	51
Other items	0.9	7.0	0.9	1.4	1.7	1.9	1.9	10	2.0	17.4	4.1	30.8	1.5	13.6	1.5	11
Total	12.8	100.0	16.0	18.7	19.6	19.9	19.7	100	11.5	100.0	13.3	100.0	10.9	100.0	13.0	100

[a] Herbertsson (161).
[b] Two sets of figures are given for 1980, owing to the use of two different methods of calculation.
[c] Hallberg (162).
[d] Arab et al. (39).
[e] Galan et al. (38).
[f] Haraldsdottir et al. (163).

increased significantly, mainly because the levels of iron fortification have been increased. Beginning in 1944, white wheat flour was fortified with iron to the normal level for whole wheat, and then with an additional 3.0 mg iron per 100 g flour. In 1963, this was increased to 5.0 mg iron per 100 g of all sifted flour, and in 1970 the level was increased to 6.5 mg iron per 100 g flour.

Studies on bioavailability suggest that about 15% of the fortification iron in Sweden is potentially available for absorption (160). To this figure is added the absorbable iron derived from food. Recent analyses made in Sweden (161) in 1984 and in Denmark in 1985 (163) show a very similar distribution of iron sources. In the Federal Republic of Germany, however, iron supplies are different (39); iron intake is higher than in Scandinavia, whether expressed in absolute terms or as the ratio of dietary iron to dietary energy. In the Federal Republic of Germany, food is not fortified with iron, but the amount of absorbable iron per unit of dietary energy is markedly higher. These figures are uncertain, however. The value of 13.3 mg per day has been derived from a 24-hour dietary recall study. A one-week study of diet gives a value 10 mg higher. These discrepancies reveal some of the problems of assessing iron intakes.

In a sample of French women (38), the prevalence of anaemia and iron deficiency were lower than in Swedish women. The French women ate more meat, fruit and vegetables — the dietary items that enhance iron absorption. Unfortunately, the women studied in France were not randomly selected, so their diet may not be representative of the whole community. However, the average yearly intake of meat in 1982 (164) was much higher in France (92 kg per year) than in Sweden (59 kg per year). French women, therefore, seem to have a significantly lower risk of developing iron deficiency than the average Scandinavian woman. The diet of women in the United Kingdom seems little better than the Scandinavian diet, since 14- and 15-year-old girls in Birmingham had similar or even lower figures for iron dietary density (4.2 mg iron per 1000 kcal) than those for the Scandinavian diet.

If the nutrient density of the diet is low, people will eat less as they become more inactive, and thereby reduce their total iron intake. This may be a further factor in the deterioration in iron status in the elderly. This, in turn, suggests that changes in diet that lead to an increase in nutrient density, such as reducing sugar and fat intakes, will help to limit the incidence of anaemia.

Folic acid intakes
Intakes of folic acid have not been measured in many European countries. Care must be taken with the analysis, since all naturally occurring folates show varying degrees of instability. The active compound pteroylmonoglutamate is formed when the extra glutamates present in natural form are removed by digestive enzymes or by an enzyme within food itself. Heat, oxidation and ultraviolet light inactivate the folate molecule, but reducing agents such as vitamin C preserve folic acid. Cooking practices can therefore affect the folic acid content of food, and the intake of folate may show seasonal increases as more vegetables are consumed. Intakes varied in Ireland from 114 µg per day in spring to 158 µg per day in winter (165). In

the United Kingdom average intakes of about 210 µg per day have been reported *(166)*. The estimated minimum requirement is 60 µg per day and recommended intakes (to cover the needs of the population) are 3.3 µg per kg body weight in men and 3.0 µg/kg in women, or about 200 µg and 170 µg per day, respectively. In Sweden, both adult men (410 µg) and the elderly (202 µg in men and 209 µg in women) meet the recommended intakes on average, but healthy adult women have a somewhat lower intake at 160 µg per day *(167,168)*. Substantially lower intakes have, however, been reported *(169,170)* from Denmark in pregnant women (82 µg), in teenage girls (70 µg) and in the elderly (52–59 µg). Perhaps only about 70% of the dietary intake of folates is actually absorbed, so deficiencies can be expected to occur in an appreciable proportion of the population. All foods of plant or animal origin contain folates, but excessive cooking can lead to substantial losses.

Goitre

An adequate intake of iodine is crucial for the prevention of goitre and the other syndromes resulting from iodine deficiency *(53)*. Compounds that interfere in one way or another with the normal uptake of iodine into the thyroid or with the metabolism of thyroidal hormones are well recognized, but they have little impact on people whose iodine intake is adequate.

Experience from countries in which iodine prophylaxis is mandatory has shown that the iodine content of salt must be at least 20 mg/kg in areas where there is little iodine in other components of the diet if the iodine intake of 150–300 µg per day recommended by WHO is to be achieved.

The overall results of the survey of iodine deficiency disorders in Europe showed a clear need for greater efforts to increase iodine intakes in countries *(53)*. The review reports on an analysis of 104 samples of commercial salt from 19 European countries. The iodine content was significantly lower than that intended by the manufacturer in 30% of the samples. Preventing iodine deficiency is straightforward and cheap, and national policy decisions on the use of iodized salt are clearly needed.

5

Strategies to help prevent major diseases

A number of themes from earlier chapters point to a common set of dietary recommendations for the prevention of many of the diseases discussed in this book. For example, evidence for the role of diet in the development of cardiovascular disease points to the need to limit saturated fatty acid intake. In many countries, this can be most readily achieved by limiting total fat intake. Measures recommended for the prevention of obesity include the suggestion that the total fat and sucrose content of the diet should fall. Both of these recommendations aim to reduce the energy density and increase the nutrient density of the diet. Of course, both children and adults would then need to adjust their intakes to cover their energy needs by eating increased amounts of starchy food. The results would be likely to benefit the general nutritional state because mineral and vitamin intakes are likely to rise, thus minimizing other nutritional problems such as iron-deficiency anaemia.

An increase in the consumption of cereals, roots, vegetables and fruit must form the main compensation for the decline in fat and sugar intakes. This would also meet the recommendation that dietary fibre intakes should increase to prevent constipation and diverticular disease; dietary potassium would also rise. These changes are likely to be particularly beneficial in the elderly and in other groups whose total energy intake is low.

A common pattern of changes in food consumption emerges from these recommendations, and one coherent plan could be produced to prevent several diseases. It is not necessary to argue for dietary change on the basis of only one dietary effect. A fall in sucrose intake, for example, has several benefits in addition to the prevention of dental caries. Nor is it necessary to propose only one way of compensating for the reduction in fat and sugar intake. The types of cereal, fruit or vegetables — or low-fat milk, meat or fish products — will obviously depend on prevailing food habits and the availability of alternative products in countries.

One way to make the proposed changes in diet in many European countries is to alter manufacturing practices to allow the provision of foods with a higher nutritional value. For example, salt intakes depend particularly on the addition of salt to products by food manufacturers. If cereal consumption is to rise, the high salt content of bread and breakfast cereals will need to fall appreciably to allow both an increase in cereal consumption and a fall in salt intake.

Community-wide and Individual Nutrient Goals

How can national and international committees define an average nutrient intake as optimum? Dietary patterns vary widely throughout Europe and within countries. Another problem arises from the need to tailor recommendations to individuals of different sex, age and physiological state (such as pregnancy or lactation). Finally, the difficulty of coping with the range of response in a group of individuals to a standardized diet is widely recognized. Should there be, therefore, a national strategy based on a single set of nutrient goals?

In theory, it is possible to envisage a single set or range of nutrient intakes that, when expressed as averages on a national basis, is associated with the minimum incidence of nutrition-related diseases, whether they result from deficiency or excess. One of the concerns in making any national nutrient recommendations, however, is that they should not be harmful. In practice, some recommendations may fail to take account of the vulnerability of specific groups within the population. For example, the original fortification policy in the United Kingdom for adding vitamin D to infant milk preparations dramatically reduced the incidence of rickets but unfortunately led to an increase in cases of hypercalcaemia from vitamin D toxicity. The level of vitamin D fortification was modified, and rickets was almost eliminated without inducing vitamin D toxicity in other children. This concept of assessing risk is important; it has constrained the development of radical policies for major change. Where vulnerable groups can be readily identified, it is easier to refine national nutrient goals to cope with the special needs of the vulnerable group than to produce goals for universal application.

Obviously, food patterns within the population vary, as does individual susceptibility to nutrition-related diseases. To work on the basis of a national average intake is therefore a very crude policy. Nevertheless, average national diets can be assessed by aggregating existing dietary data and relating them to national disease patterns. This is the first step in developing national nutrient recommendations and for monitoring the rate of change towards national dietary goals. Expert committees should choose each goal, aiming for appreciable benefit with the minimum of risk. In addition to these national averages, some central governments and health and educational services are now attempting to refine nutritional goals to make them appropriate to state, regional or, indeed, individual needs.

Nutrient Goals

What nutrient goals would help prevent, for example, cardiovascular disease? Two WHO groups *(12,94)* make certain recommendations for countries with a high incidence of coronary heart disease. These countries should:

— reduce average cholesterol concentrations to less than 5.17 mmol/litre (200 mg/dl) by reducing saturated fat intake to less than 10% of total energy intake, reducing dietary cholesterol to less than 300 mg per day, and avoiding obesity;

— reduce average blood pressure by reducing salt intake to less than 5 g per day, controlling obesity and avoiding excess alcohol intake;

— avoid smoking;

— increase exercise, to avoid obesity, and reduce blood pressure and blood cholesterol;

— avoid softening community water supplies; and

— introduce measures for the whole population, starting in childhood.

The recommendations developed by WHO expert committees and scientific groups are not new. This is shown in Table 20, which lists the recommendations of many international bodies *(171)*. Given the remarkable uniformity of these recommendations, there seems to be no need to develop a distinctive set of goals for the European Region. The WHO Expert Committee on Prevention of Coronary Heart Disease *(94)* suggests that an ideal mean serum cholesterol concentration might be 4.14 mmol/litre (160 mg/dl) for adults and 2.85 mmol/litre (110 mg/dl) for children aged 5–18 years. Further, low rates of atherosclerosis and coronary heart disease are possible when the dietary fat amounts to as little as 10% of the energy intake (as in Japan) or as much as 40% (as in Crete, where diets are high in monounsaturated fatty acids). Provided that the saturated fat intake is less than 10% and polyunsaturated fat 3% or more of the daily energy intake, rates of coronary heart disease are low. On this basis, the Committee recommended an ideal goal for saturated fatty acids of 10% of total energy, with total fat intake amounting to 20–30% of total energy.

Population Strategy or High-risk Strategy?

The same Expert Committee *(94)* set out the reasons for establishing a population approach, as well as for a high-risk strategy. Is there additional evidence to support a population approach in Europe? Fig. 37, from the Framingham study, shows that the distribution of serum cholesterol within a population at high risk of coronary heart disease is so wide that more people with an average level of serum cholesterol die of coronary heart disease than those at high risk *(172)*. This estimate depends, however, on the lack of an observed threshold in serum cholesterol below which coronary heart disease rates are not reduced. It has been argued, however, on the basis of data from the Pooling Project *(173)*, that serum cholesterol need not fall below about 5.14 mmol/litre (200 mg/dl) in adults because no further benefit accrues. This in turn means that, if there are worries about reducing existing cholesterol levels because of hypothetical changes in membrane chemistry, a policy of population screening to identify the high-risk group is preferable *(174)*.

Fortunately, European evidence (Fig. 30) shows a progressive fall in risk down to the lowest ranking of serum cholesterol. The Gothenburg men *(77)*

Table 20. Early recommendations of 18 scientific and medical committees on dietary fats and coronary heart disease

Country and committee	Date	Target group	Percentage of total energy derived from fat	Increased intake of polyunsaturated fat	P:S ratio	Daily dietary cholesterol (mg)	Reduction of sugar	Labelling of fat content
Norway, Sweden and Finland	1968	GP[a]	25–35	Yes	—	—	Yes	Yes
United States, Inter-Society	1970	GP HR[b]	<35	Yes	1.0	<300	—	Yes
New Zealand, Heart Foundation	1971	GP HR	35 35	— Yes	— 1.0	300–600 300–600	No No	Yes Yes
New Zealand, Royal Society	1971	GP HR	Avoid excess saturated fat	No Yes	— —	Reduce Reduce	— —	— —
United States, American Health Foundation	1972	GP	35	Yes	1.0	300	Yes	Yes
United States, American Medical Association	1972	HR	Substantial decrease in saturated fat	Yes	—	Reduce	—	Yes
International Society of Cardiology	1973	HR	<30	Yes	>1.0	<300	—	Yes
Netherlands	1973	GP	35	Yes	1.0	250–300	Yes	Yes
United States, American Heart Association	1973	GP	35	Yes	1.0	300	Yes	Yes

United States, White House Conference	1973	GP	35	Yes	—	300	—	Yes
Australia, National Heart Foundation	1974	GP	30–35	Yes	1.5	<300	—	—
		HR	30–35	Yes	1.5	<300	Yes	—
United Kingdom, Department of Health and Social Security, COMA report	1974	GP	Reduce total fat, especially saturated fat	No	—	—	Yes	Yes
Australia, Academy of Science	1975	GP	35	Yes	1.0	<350	Yes	Yes
Federal Republic of Germany	1975	GP	Reduce saturated fat	Yes	—	300	—	—
Canada, Department of Health and Welfare	1976	GP	30–35	Yes	—	400	Yes	Yes
		HR	30–35	Yes	—	400	Yes	Yes
New Zealand, Royal Society	1976	GP	Decrease saturated fat	Yes	Increase	Reduce	—	—
Norway, Ministry of Agriculture	1976	GP	35	Yes	—	—	Yes	Yes
United Kingdom, Royal College of Physicians, & British Cardiac Society	1976	GP	Towards 35	Yes	—	Reduce	Yes	Yes
United States, Senate Committee	1977	GP	30	Yes	1.0	300	Yes	Yes
		HR	30	Yes	1.0	300	Yes	Yes

[a] General population.

[b] High-risk group.

Source: Dietary fats and oils in human nutrition (171).

Fig. 37. Prevalence distribution (histogram) of serum cholesterol concentrations related to coronary heart disease mortality in men aged 55-64 years

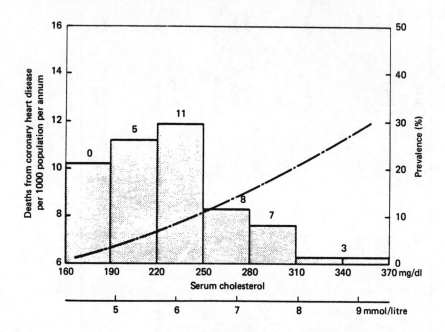

Note. The interrupted line represents mortality from coronary heart disease, and the number above each column represents an estimate of deaths attributed to this condition per 1000 population per ten-year period.

Source: Kannel & Gordon *(172)*.

showed, as did the Framingham men *(172)*, a progressive rise in risk with increasing levels of cholesterol. These data resemble the older findings of Keys et al. *(73)*, who also found, on a cross-cultural basis, a good relationship between serum cholesterol and coronary heart disease at all levels of circulating cholesterol.

Even if countries adopt a single set of nutrient goals, however, it is not possible for all countries to achieve them within the next 10-15 years. Different countries have therefore developed their own nutrient goals, so that the direction of change can be established. Table 21 summarizes recent national nutrient goals proposed by expert committees in four countries. All emphasize the total population approach.

106

Table 21. National nutrient goals in four countries

	Norway, 1975		Sweden, 1983	Great Britain, 1984		Netherlands, 1986
	General population	High-risk group	General population (by the year 2000)	General population	High-risk group[a]	General population
Percentage of total energy derived from:						
sugar	10%		Reduce to 10%[b]	No increase		Total mono- and disaccharides. 15–25%
total fat	35	35	30	35	30	30–35
saturated fat			—	15	10	Reduce
P:S ratio	0.5	1.0	0.5	0.45		0.5–1.0
Cholesterol (mg/1000 kcal)		Reduce	—	No recommendation	<100	No increase; currently 138
Salt (g/day)			≦8	—		≦9
Fibre (g/day)			30–35	Increase	>30	Increase by 25% to 3 g/MJ
Protein	No change			No change		No change
Alcohol consumption			Limit	Limit		Limit
Maintain ideal weight[c]	Yes	Yes	Yes	Yes	Yes	Yes
Labelling			Yes	Yes		Yes

[a] Potassium-rich foods for people on diuretic therapy.

[b] The figure of 10% is obtained by difference since a starch intake of 45–50% is recommended and lactose (about 5%) is excluded from the refined sugar figure.

[c] Ideal weight is frequently identified as a BMI of 20–25.

These goals reflect the wish for the development of preventive measures that are consistent with the ability of the agricultural industry in each country to adapt. For instance, an attempt in Scandinavian countries to decrease, within a comparatively short time, the national average intake of saturated fatty acids to only 10% of total energy intake would have grave effects on farming. Without dramatic and impracticable changes in the breeds of animals and a total change in animal husbandry, butchery and marketing techniques, large numbers of people would have to shift to a specific form of vegetarianism to allow the saturated fat intake to fall sufficiently. The price of dairy produce might also change drastically if low-fat milk (0.5% fat) were universally drunk and butter were no longer commonly used. Many expert committees, recognizing the economic problems of too rapid a change, have settled for more modest proposals, which a responsive population could achieve and which would allow adjustment of the structure of the agricultural industry.

The development of intermediate targets for some European countries is therefore realistic. The national recommendations differ only in minor ways. The Swedish guidelines are based on a broad view of a preventive nutritional policy, while those for Great Britain were exclusively linked to the prevention of cardiovascular diseases. This may explain the enigmatic statement by the British committee that sugar intakes should not increase; the Swedish committee advocates a figure of 10% dietary energy from sugar. The Obesity Working Party of the Royal College of Physicians (56) advocated halving sugar intakes in the United Kingdom, which would bring them into line with the Swedish goals. The recent Dutch nutrient goals (175) suggest a figure of 15–25% for all monosaccharides and disaccharides (including lactose, which probably provides about 5% of energy). Given the natural simple sugar content of fruits and vegetables, this implies a very substantial reduction in the amount of simple sugars added to manufactured food products.

Table 1 (p. xii) suggests a common set of goals. They may be considered suitable for many European countries. Nations that have not developed their own goals could find these helpful. Obviously, in several countries, excessive intakes of sucrose or saturated fatty acids will not be considered a problem. Under such circumstances, government nutrition policy objectives need to be based on the ultimate goals, with their emphasis on the ideal figures for national intakes of fat, saturated fatty acid and sucrose.

Combining a High-risk Strategy with a Population Strategy

The WHO recommendations on the prevention of cardiovascular disease (94) involve approaches aimed at both the population and people at high risk. The two approaches are complementary; a greater change in diet is advocated for people at greater risk. The recent report from the Committee on Medical Aspects of Food Policy (5) takes a similar approach.

A few experts continue to argue that the population approach is ill conceived, that only people at high risk should alter their diets. This approach is strongly advocated by some physicians trained and experienced in

108

the management of individual patients. With a medical practice dominated by the treatment of disease and the evident benefits of tailoring a patient's management to his or her individual needs, some physicians have difficulty in seeing a public health problem in epidemiological terms. For some diseases, a strategy of prevention for the high-risk group may be particularly important. Ideally, each medical condition, particularly hypertension or obesity, should be considered on its own to see whether both the population and the high-risk strategies are needed. Unfortunately, only limited analyses have been made of these alternatives, and present recommendations are largely confined to limiting coronary heart disease and high blood pressure. Clearly, governments would be wise to regard both the population and the high-risk approaches as necessary.

The high-risk strategy
There is some debate as to how best to apply preventive measures to a population and how to include a high-risk strategy. Should the middle-aged population, or perhaps younger age groups, be screened to identify people at high risk of developing major diseases? Mass screening as a measure to prevent coronary heart disease is theoretically possible; identifying risk factors to prevent hypertension, obesity, osteoporosis and diverticular disease, however, is difficult without the use of the individual's family history as a basis for action. In addition, screening could identify people with medium risk from a high normal blood pressure or BMI or a relatively low bone density.

As a further attempt to refine the high-risk strategy, it is possible to take a dietary approach, identifying the people whose diet does not conform to the guidelines and then providing them with advice on how to change it. The Committee on Medical Aspects of Food Policy advocated this approach *(5)* and it has led to the use of simple, if inaccurate, techniques for assessing the diet of individuals within the population. In addition, it neglects the varying genetic susceptibility of different individuals within the population. Thus, such screening would not identify very reactive people with a dietary saturated fat intake just below the specified upper limit (14% of total energy intake), although changes in diet would be deemed necessary for non-reactive children and adults whose saturated fat intake was 16% of total energy.

These examples emphasize the dilemma faced by policy-makers, who must consider the overall impact of their proposals. High-risk strategies should be considered to amplify the work of population strategies, which aim to change the distribution of risk factors. The costs of, and opportunities for, screening and follow-up action need to be taken into account.

The population approach
The population approach has been considered in some detail by the WHO Scientific Group on Primary Prevention of Essential Hypertension *(12)* and in the recent report of the WHO Expert Committee on Community Prevention and Control of Cardiovascular Diseases *(176)*. The argument for a preventive effort has also been considered by the Faculty of Community Medicine of the Royal College of Physicians in the United Kingdom.

Preventing hypertension
Preventing hypertension is clearly preferable to treating it but has received much less attention from the medical profession. Rose *(177)* has pointed out large numbers of deaths in people with mildly elevated blood pressure. As risk increases progressively from the lowest to the highest blood pressure level, achieving a modest reduction in those with mild elevations of blood pressure is likely to benefit more people than limiting preventive and therapeutic attention to those with extreme hypertension. It has been calculated in Sweden, for example, that a 10 mmHg reduction in the population's average blood pressure would prevent as much morbidity as reducing the blood pressure of all hypertensives to the normal range *(178)*. In the United Kingdom, Marmot *(179)* has suggested that a reduction of only 4 mmHg in mean blood pressure in the population would result in a 9% fall in mortality from coronary heart disease and a 20% drop in cerebrovascular mortality. It is thus not surprising that the WHO Scientific Group on Primary Prevention of Essential Hypertension *(13)* concluded that a population approach to the prevention of hypertension was desirable. The Group also specified an excess of energy, alcohol and salt in the diet as major factors in the pathogenesis of hypertension and indicated that weight maintenance and a reduction in saturated fat intake could be desirable.

The same argument applies here as in the prevention of coronary heart disease: a small change in the average value for a risk factor of a whole population, such as blood pressure, is likely to be of greater benefit than a preventive strategy aimed at a high-risk group.

Treating hypertension
Many studies have shown that about half the hypertensives in a country are undiagnosed. Of the diagnosed hypertensives, only about half are actually treated for their condition, and poor results are achieved in half of those who receive drug therapy. Therefore, perhaps only one eighth of hypertensives are treated adequately. In addition, Stamler et al.[a] have noted that drug treatment of mild hypertension may have risks that outweigh the benefits. The risks not only include the increased likelihood of heart arrythmias, with excessive losses of urinary potassium, but also result from the drugs used. These drugs increase the risk factors for coronary heart disease; they increase levels of plasma total cholesterol, low-density lipoprotein cholesterol, very-low-density lipoprotein cholesterol and triglycerides, and they lower levels of high-density lipoprotein cholesterol *(180)*. A change in diet is therefore needed simply to limit the disadvantageous effects of the drugs on lipid metabolism. Drug treatment is also costly, in terms of both the drugs and the personnel required to monitor the treatment.

The more detailed and sustained dietary advice given to the hypertensives studied in the Multiple Risk Factor Intervention Trial *(84)* led to an

---

[a] **Stamler, J. et al.** *High blood pressure: role in coronary heart disease and implications for prevention and control.* Geneva, World Health Organization, 1983 (unpublished document WHO/CVD/83.5).

appreciable reduction in lipid risk factors despite the use of oral diuretics. One of the important determinants of benefit seemed to be the need for a moderate weight loss in those individuals who were about 5 kg above their appropriate weight. Weight loss limited both the increases in blood glucose and uric acid resulting from the use of diuretics and the adverse effects of beta-blockers on plasma lipids. There is also increasing evidence that nutritional changes can be an important adjunct of drug treatment (181).

Stamler et al.[a] suggested the following guidelines for the management of mild hypertension. First, much more attention should be given to non-pharmacological nutritional and hygienic approaches to lower less severe high blood pressure. When these alone do not suffice and drug prescription is indicated, nutritional and hygienic measures should be continued (to minimize the number of drugs and dosages needed), along with special attention to nutritional aspects to minimize drug complications. High-dose diuretics should be avoided in less severe hypertensives, and particularly in those with electrocardiographic abnormalities. Finally, nutritional and hygienic recommendations should be included in the long-term control of all major risk factors, particularly hypercholesterolaemia and cigarette smoking. The combination of effects is likely to contribute to reducing the probability of morbidity and mortality from coronary heart disease in people with hypertension.

Hypertensive trials are difficult to evaluate from a nutritional point of view because cardiologists and epidemiologists focus so much of their attention on managing blood pressure with drugs rather than dietary change or alterations in other aspects of lifestyle. Nevertheless, on many occasions overweight has been shown to be an extremely important determinant of the prevalence of high blood pressure in a community. An excess body weight in young adult life, with a further increase in weight, is particularly likely to lead to the development of hypertension.

Recent studies from Chicago (182) showed that 59% of hypertensive men and women who were given nutritional advice (to reduce weight, modify fat intake, lower salt intake and avoid heavy alcohol consumption) responded and maintained normal blood pressure without needing any further medication. Such reductions in blood pressure have been sustained for up to four years (183) and other benefits, such as lower levels of serum cholesterol, have been obtained.

One study, involving a high-risk group of men aged 40–59 years, with diastolic blood pressure of 80–89 mmHg, showed that changes in diet, the avoidance of cigarette smoking and an increase in isotonic exercise led to a sustained but moderate weight loss and reductions in both systolic and diastolic blood pressure that were maintained for almost a decade. Blood pressure is usually expected to increase in men of this age (183).

These findings imply that adults with very modest increases in diastolic blood pressure will benefit from modifying their diet and exercise patterns. If generally applicable, this regimen would therefore be relevant for the

---

[a] Ibid.

approximately two thirds of the European male population with diastolic blood pressure over 80 mmHg. Clearly, such a policy of prevention could not be implemented by health professionals but requires a public health policy for the whole population. The evidence of clinical trials seems to amplify the epidemiological evidence of the benefits of preventing high blood pressure.

Approaches to the Prevention of Certain Conditions

No clear assessment has yet been made as to whether a high-risk strategy, in addition to a population approach, helps to prevent cancer or obesity. The risk of cancer is not readily identifiable in subgroups of the population and the risk factors are in any case uncertain. In obesity, a plethora of conditions seem to lead to morbidity as well as to an increased risk of death as weight is gained. Recently, many people have wished to reduce the anxiety of people who are only mildly overweight since their risk of death may be no greater than those of an acceptable weight. Only in grade 2 obesity (a BMI over 30) does the mortality risk begin to increase rapidly. This distinction between mild and moderate obesity may be appropriate for individual physicians, who can assess the risks of hypertension, hypercholesterolaemia and diabetes in their patients, but a population strategy should advocate measures that encourage the maintenance of weight within the acceptable range throughout adult life. This would seem to be the best policy for limiting the morbidity, as well as the mortality, associated with obesity.

Population strategies for specific age groups?

The recommendations presented so far suggest a general population approach to prevention. It could be argued, however, that such an approach is appropriate only for young and middle-aged adults, on the grounds that children or the elderly have special needs.

Young children

A recent British report on the prevention of cardiovascular diseases (5) has advised that the recommendations made should not be applied to children aged less than 5 years. The choice of low-fat milk, for example, could lead to an inappropriate diet for young children, who depend on milk. In the United States, however, a recent consensus conference on heart disease (184)considered the general dietary measures recommended to be appropriate for children aged over 2 years. Elsewhere in Europe children have not been specifically excluded from dietary recommendations. Obviously, great care must be taken when babies transfer to weaning diets from a dependence on breast-milk, in which fat makes up 50% of total energy. Each community will need to develop its own policy, consistent with its cultural patterns of child-rearing. The key nutritional factor is the need to keep milk of normal fat content in the child's diet until most of the energy intake comes from food other than milk. Changing to milk with a very low fat content too early in life means that babies obtain excessive amounts of sodium as they consume more milk in an effort to satisfy energy needs.

The elderly

Life expectancy is increasing at a remarkable rate in the elderly, but it is less certain that the quality of life matches its length. Present data suggest that the number of years through which the elderly suffer from physical, mental and social disability is tending to increase, so the increase in survival is accompanied by more years of ill health *(185)*. Women tend to live longer with diminishing functional abilities than men. In the United Kingdom, chronic ill health limits the activities of 41% of people aged 65–74 years and 60% of those over 85.

A recent review by WHO[a] of the nutritional needs of the elderly concluded that the dietary recommendations suggested for young and middle-aged adults were equally appropriate for older people. As energy intakes decline in response to reduced physical activity, the chances of nutritional deficiencies will increase progressively. An increase in the nutrient density of the diets of the elderly would thus be advantageous. The maintenance of physical activity is also a major consideration; it may do a great deal to enhance an old person's sense of wellbeing and lead to an increase in food intake. Elderly people should not therefore be excluded from dietary recommendations; they may have as much, or more, to gain as the rest of the community. Nevertheless, many of their chronic physical and mental problems are of unknown origin and require more research *(185)*.

Weight reduction, however, should not be routinely advocated for the elderly. Undoubtedly, many people with a variety of medical conditions (such as angina, hiatus hernia, arthritis, or simple breathlessness) would benefit from weight reduction, but there is little evidence to justify a health education campaign aiming to reduce the BMI of the whole elderly population to the range considered suitable for young and middle-aged adults. This does not mean, however, that adults should not avoid gaining weight as they age.

[a] *Nutrition in the elderly.* Copenhagen, WHO Regional Office for Europe, 1987 (unpublished document IRP/HEE 114.2.5).

113

6

Do nutrient patterns match up to WHO and national recommendations?

Is the type of food eaten in many European countries conducive to good health? Evidence shows marked variations in the Region, both in the type of food eaten and in the patterns of nutrition-related diseases. The evidence on the nutritional origin of these diseases has come from studies assessing the roles of individual nutrients rather than foods.

Hypotheses about atheroma and saturated fats have thus developed from epidemiological studies such as the work of Keys *(70)*. Such hypotheses have been amplified by metabolic, human and animal research to identify possible mechanisms and thereby allow greater confidence in conclusions about the desirable intake of specific nutrients such as saturated fat. Some additional epidemiological studies link the consumption of particular foods,· not nutrients, with disease. This evidence is much less reliable because it can only provide clues to the mechanisms involved.

In developing objectives for nutrition policies, expert committees have therefore concentrated on evidence on nutrient rather than food intake. The extent of the changes needed becomes clear in the light of differences between the nutrient patterns of individual countries and the nutrient goals for the prevention of cardiovascular disease and other conditions.

Dietary Fat Intake

Fig. 38 shows information on the fat content of diets in European countries in 1980, expressed in terms of the energy content of the diet from all sources except alcohol. The figures shown are crude averages for the whole country: there may be marked differences between regions of a country as well as within the population. For example, studies in Moscow and Leningrad show that fat consumption in men aged 40–59 years is about 38% of total energy intake *(186)*. The actual average food supply for the whole of the Asian and European regions of the USSR, however, corresponds to an optimal intake as defined by WHO. Countries have been listed in ascending order. Only five countries meet the ultimate WHO goal for fat intake. A further three fall

Fig. 38. Estimated percentage of total energy derived from fat in some European countries

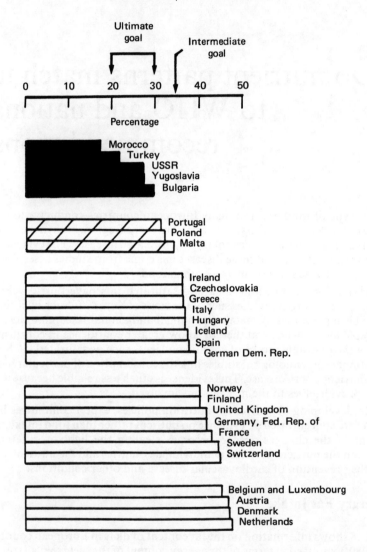

Source: Food balance sheets, 1979–81 average (3).

below the proposed intermediate goals. Countries with a low proportion of energy suplies derived from fat are located in either the Mediterranean area or eastern Europe. It is northern and western European countries in which fat intake makes up more than 40% of dietary energy. Thus, the geographical differences in food consumption are repeated in data on nutrients. Fig. 39 shows the total fat content in diets in Europe.

The fluctuating intakes of total fat and saturated fat over a 25-year period in Norway and Sweden are shown in Fig. 40. In Sweden, total fat consumption decreased substantially from 1970 to 1973, perhaps reflecting the impact of the national diet and exercise campaign started in 1970. In 1973, however, the Swedish Ministry of Agriculture introduced subsidies on a variety of fat-enriched products for economic rather than health reasons. By this time, the Norwegians were developing their national nutrition policy and the role of diet in health became of much greater interest. Whether these government and other preventive initiatives led to the observed changes in diet cannot be proved, but the data suggest that the intakes of saturated and total fat in a population can change appreciably in a short period.

The picture is not static. Even in a country such as Bulgaria, with a total fat supply within the ideal range, the fat content of the diet has increased progressively. There seems to have been a progressive trend towards increased intake in most European countries over the last 15 years. This trend seems to have stabilized a bit since 1980, but this has resulted mainly from the maintenance or decline of fat availability in countries where fat intake is already very high (Austria, Iceland, Ireland, the Netherlands and Norway). Only in Portugal and Romania does dietary fat appear to remain stable at an appropriate level.

Although the proportion of energy derived from fat has increased in almost every country in Europe over the last 35 years, this does not always represent an absolute increase in the total fat content of the diet. In the United Kingdom, for example, household surveys show that the total amount of fat purchased has hardly changed at all. Carbohydrate intake has declined steadily, however, as suggested by the fall in the consumption of cereals, roots and tubers noted earlier. A fall in carbohydrate intake automatically means a rise in the proportion of energy derived from fat.

There is a weak relationship between the total fat content of diets in countries and the rate of coronary heart disease. This is not surprising; saturated fat is more important than total fat in the development of this disease.

Saturated fat intakes
In Fig. 41, the rate of mortality from ischaemic heart disease in men aged 35–64 years is plotted against the estimated average national supply of saturated fat. Of course, the figures are based on food supplies, not actual intakes, and do not take account of different cooking or manufacturing practices. Fig. 41 simply indicates the range of saturated fat supplies and should not be seen to refute the hypotheses on diet and heart disease. The relationship shown is not statistically significant.

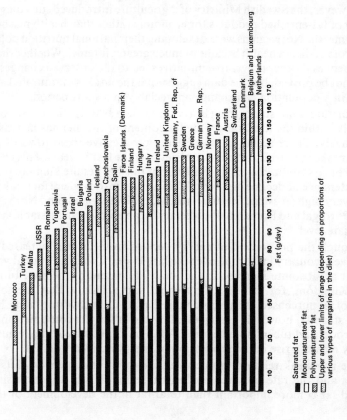

Fig. 39. Average fat supplies in diets in European countries

Note. Where the sources of margarine are unspecified then two values for margarines (one assuming a high saturated fat content, the other with a low saturated fat content) have been calculated; the effects of this range are shown.

Source: Food balance sheets, 1979–81 average (3).

Fig. 40. Fat intakes in Norway and Sweden, 1960–1985

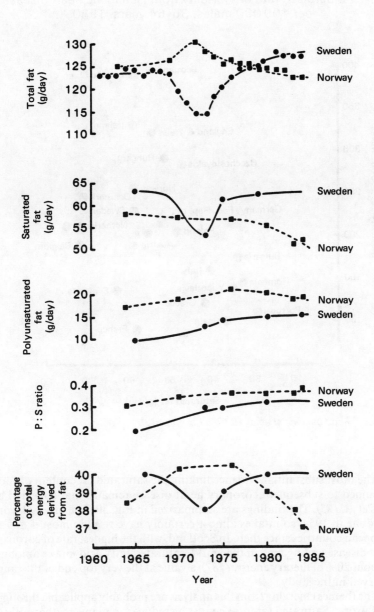

Source: Isaksson, B. (personal communication).

119

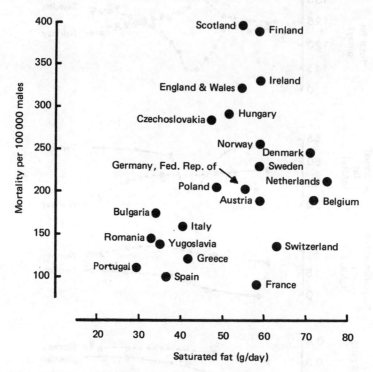

Fig. 41. The relationship of saturated fat supplies to the standardized rate of mortality from ischaemic heart disease per 100 000 males, 35–64 years, 1980

Source: Food balance sheets, 1979–81 average (3).

The most substantial evidence linking the saturated fat content of food consumed to subsequent coronary heart disease remains that collected by Keys et al. *(73)*. The findings are summarized in Fig. 30. The original work was done in 1954, so intakes almost certainly have risen in most if not all European countries since then. In Scotland, with the highest rate of coronary heart disease among men in the world, saturated fatty acid intake amounts to about 20% of dietary energy *(187)*, a value at the very top end of the range observed in the study.

The themes emerging from this analysis are probably applicable throughout Europe. Saturated fat intake must be reduced in many northern European communities. Countries in eastern Europe need to arrest and indeed reverse their current trends towards increased saturated fat intakes. Mediterranean countries need to guard against changes in diet that might lead towards the northern European pattern of eating.

120

Sources of total fat and saturated fat in the European diet
Fat is derived from many sources; only when the sources in each country are recognized can reasonable national food and health policy objectives be developed.

Some information about the sources of fat in the diets in different European countries can be gained from FAO food balance sheets. Some countries provide additional information from household food surveys. Fig. 42 and 43, as illustrations, show the proportions of saturated fat derived from different sources in the British and Italian diets. The British data are derived from a British household food consumption survey (1980); the Italian figures are recalculated from food balance data. It is clear that dairy products and meat provide the major input in Great Britain *(188)*, with vegetable oils contributing only a small amount. In Italy *(189)*, the position is very different; vegetable fats contribute a greater proportion of the total fat intake than animal fats. Of course, vegetable oils as such cannot automatically be assumed to be low in saturated fat, but this is likely to be true in Italy because of the high contribution of olive oil to the vegetable fats used.

Fig. 42. Sources of saturated fat in the British diet

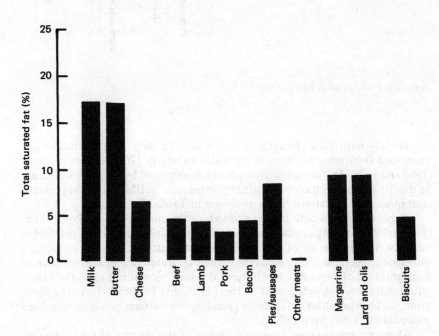

Source: Walker *(188)*.

121

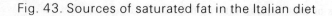

Fig. 43. Sources of saturated fat in the Italian diet

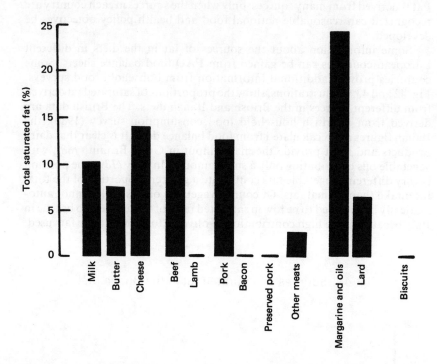

Source: Ferro-Luzzi & Sette *(189)*.

Dietary habits are changing quite rapidly. In Italy, total fat intake has increased substantially, from 90 g per day to nearly 120 g per day between 1965 and 1979. Animal fat consumption has increased by 40%. This increase in dietary fat has been accompanied by an increase in BMI, in blood pressure and in serum cholesterol *(190)*, as shown in Table 22.

Table 23 gives a detailed breakdown of the changes in the Polish diet. Total edible fat consumption has increased very substantially, with a larger increase in the intake of vegetable oil than butter. Natural as well as processed vegetable oils can be very high in saturated fat, and the increasing consumption of vegetable and butter fat is now recognized to be the major disadvantageous development in the Polish diet (Table 24). At the same time, the consumption of fats from cereals (predominantly polyunsaturated essential fats), has been halved.

These examples show how assessments of the sources of fat in the diet can be used to begin the development of a rational scheme for adjusting government policy and, in consequence, food and agricultural practices. Fig. 42 shows that about 25% of the saturated fat in Britain is derived from

122

Table 22. Changes in coronary risk factors and
myocardial infarction in two groups of Italian men
aged 51–59 years

	1965 (N = 593)	1975 (N = 553)
Serum cholesterol level (mmol/litre)	5.23	5.75
Systolic blood pressure (mmHg)	148	147
Diastolic blood pressure (mmHg)	86	89
Cigarettes (per day)	7.7	7.3
BMI (kg/m²)	25.2	26.1
Physical activity at work[a]	2.6	2.4
Myocardial infarction	28	31

[a] Score: 1 = sedentary;   2 = moderate;   3 = heavy.

Source: Menotti et al. *(190)*.

meat and meat products, while dairy products provide over 40% of the total. Inevitably, therefore, the saturated fat intake from both dairy fat and meat fat must be reduced. This does not mean that the consumption of milk, cheese and meat needs to be reduced; low-fat varieties must be provided.

The economic and nutritional implications of this change need to be considered carefully. Butter is already stockpiled in western Europe, and further adjustments in agricultural economic policy are clearly needed. Care must be taken to ensure that a shift in consumption from butter to margarine does not simply substitute one form of saturated fatty acid for another.

Dietary Salt Intake

Salt intakes can be assessed directly by a variety of methods (including national statistics, questionnaires and detailed weighed intakes) or indirectly by measuring the total amount of sodium excreted in the urine over 24 hours.

Table 25 shows the mean urinary sodium output in some western societies as collated by Isaksson *(191)*, further data being obtained from a recent series of coordinated collections of urine over 24 hours from non-randomly selected subjects in different part of Europe *(192)*. The greater salt intake of the men may in part reflect their greater total food intake. The data must be treated with caution; it would be unwise to assume, on the basis of these data, that Swedish salt intakes have risen. Other analyses *(191)* suggest that sodium intakes peaked in 1975 and then fell until 1980, and that urinary sodium excretion in Belgium and in Finland (North Karelia) has declined. A renal sodium excretion of 175 mmol corresponds to a total salt intake of

Table 23. Changes in the sources of energy in Poland, 1950–1983

	Year				
	1950	1960	1970	1980	1983
Percentage of total energy derived from:					
protein	10.7	10.6	10.5	10.8	10.5
fat	21.2	25.3	29.3	33.0	31.0
carbohydrate	68.1	64.1	60.2	56.2	58.5
Percentage of total dietary protein derived from:					
animal protein	40.3	46.6	53.4	58.8	57.2
Percentage of total energy derived from:					
animal products	24.9	29.0	32.5	36.5	34.9
vegetable products	75.1	71.0	67.5	63.5	65.1

Source: unpublished data from the Food and Nutrition Institute, Warsaw, based on food balance statistics.

Table 24. Changes in the percentage contribution of different foods to total fat consumption in Poland, 1950–1983

	Year				
	1950	1960	1970	1980	1983
Cereals, including rice	10.9	8.0	5.9	4.9	5.2
Meat and offal	24.0	23.2	23.5	27.8	24.3
Fish and fish products	0.3	0.7	0.7	0.8	0.8
Milk and milk products	27.1	24.9	23.3	19.7	23.2
Hens' eggs	2.1	2.2	2.3	2.4	2.4
Total edible fats	34.0	39.4	42.9	43.3	42.8
animal fats	18.7	18.5	16.7	14.0	13.4
vegetable fats	5.3	9.2	14.0	14.0	13.5
butter	10.0	11.7	12.2	15.3	15.9

Source: unpublished data from the Food and Nutrition Institute, Warsaw, based on food balance statistics.

Table 25. Mean urinary sodium output in European populations

Country	Mean urinary sodium ouput (mmol/day)	
	Males	Females
Belgium	143	—
Belgium[a]	195	—
Denmark	—	126
Finland (North Karelia)	190	119
Finland (North Karelia)[a]	222	175
France	208	119
Germany, Federal Republic of	172	165
Germany, Federal Republic of[a]	194	—
Greece	175	139
Ireland	147	124
Italy	187	154
Netherlands	178	144
Portugal	195	153
Sweden	192	139
Sweden[a]	167	128

[a] These data are based on single 24-hour urine specimens from representative population groups *(191)* and were collected 5–10 years ago. The rest of the data are from 50 subjects of each sex, non-randomly selected from convenient groups such as laboratory workers, in different countries, and comprise the results of part of the European Community concerted action project in nutrition.

Source: Isaksson *(191)*, and Knuiman, J.T. (personal communication).

about 11 g per day and an output of 144 mmol to about 9 g per day, some sodium being excreted by routes other than urine. It seems reasonable to conclude that European adults of both sexes are eating approximately twice the 5 g salt per day that WHO considered as a goal for national averages.

Statistics are readily available from five countries in which attempts have been made to derive values for salt intakes from different sources. Table 26 classifies the salt in terms of discretionary and nondiscretionary sources. Discretionary sources include table and cooking salt, which the consumer can readily control. The data suggest that natural sources make up 1–1.5 g of salt consumed daily. Given a total intake of 9–14 g per head per day, this source therefore provides only 7–13% of total intake. It is now apparent that, although the amount of cooking salt used in the home is substantial, only a small proportion of it is actually eaten, the rest being thrown away in cooking water. Thus, when 24-hour urinary measurements of sodium are made to check on total salt intake, only about 9 g is ingested; 85% of this is

Table 26. Estimates of the proportion of dietary salt derived from different sources in different countries

Country	Salt consumption (grams per head per day)[a]					Reference
	Total	Natural	Processing	Catering	Table and cooking	
Finland[b]	12.1	1.6 (13)	5.3 (44)		5.2 (43)	193
Finland[b]	13.7			8.7 (64)	5.0 (37)	194
Finland[c]	8.6	1.1 (13)	3.8 (44)		3.7 (43)	193
Finland[c]	9.7			6.0 (62)	3.7 (38)	194
Finland	12.6	1.5 (12)	5.3 (42)	1.0 (8)	4.8 (38)	195
Sweden	11.0	1.0 (9)	5.3 (48)		4.8 (44)	196
United Kingdom	9.7	0.9 (9)	5.6 (58)		3.1 (32)	197
United Kingdom	11.7	8.1[d] (69)		1.6[d] (14)	2.0[d] (17)	179
United States	14.5		8.0 (55)		6.5 (45)	198

[a] Figures in parentheses represent percentages of total intake.

[b] Figures for men only.

[c] Figures for women only.

[d] Marmot included some cooking salt in his figures derived from Bull & Buss (197) for food consumed at home, but added values only for catering salt and table salt use as indicated to give a total value of 11.7 g per head per day.

derived from nondiscretionary sources. Table salt accounts for about 9% of salt intake and cooking salt accounts for the remaining 6% *(199)*.

Implications of analyses of salt intakes

This new information suggests that changing manufacturing practices is the most important measure to be taken in reducing salt intake. Reducing the use of table and cooking salt will also help, but not nearly as much.

This change will not be easy. Salt has a number of useful properties in food, and the taste, flavour, consistency, appearance and keeping qualities of food may all be affected by reducing its salt content. Extensive technological research may therefore be needed.

Dietary Sugar Intakes

Fig. 44 compares the sugar supplies of European countries in 1980 with the recommendation that consumption should account for 10% of total energy intake. Intakes of sugar are clearly excessive in many countries. The figures are based on national food balance sheets (which are, again, subject to error), and there is little information on individual dietary intakes with which to compare them. Dietary surveys employing a variety of techniques fail to obtain a complete record of sugar consumed in the form of confectionery. The frequency and the form of sugar intake is important for the prevention of dental caries, but data on the pattern of sugar intakes in different populations is very limited. Nevertheless, national committees have found total sugar supplies to be undesirable, as high sugar consumption contributes to reducing the nutrient and increasing the energy density of the diet. In response to concerns about obesity, people increasingly favour sugar substitutes, but there are no figures on their consumption in different European countries.

Dietary Alcohol Intakes

Fig. 45 shows the range of alcohol available for consumption in different European countries. There are no clear quantitative European guidelines, although experts in the United Kingdom have suggested a figure of 4% of total energy as the upper limit of national averages. Clearly, some countries exceed this value substantially. Alcohol consumption differs markedly among European countries, and is steadily increasing in some nations (Fig. 46).

127

Fig. 44. Estimated percentage of total energy (including alcohol) derived from sugar in some European countries

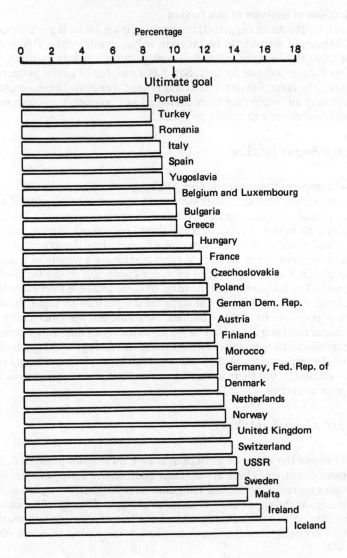

Source: Food balance sheets, 1979–81 average (3).

Fig. 45. Estimated percentage of total energy derived from alcohol in some European countries

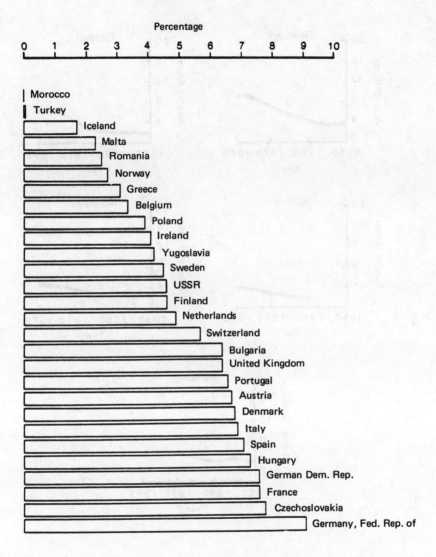

Percentage

Morocco
Turkey
Iceland
Malta
Romania
Norway
Greece
Belgium
Poland
Ireland
Yugoslavia
Sweden
USSR
Finland
Netherlands
Switzerland
Bulgaria
United Kingdom
Portugal
Austria
Denmark
Italy
Spain
Hungary
German Dem. Rep.
France
Czechoslovakia
Germany, Fed. Rep. of

Source: Food balance sheets, 1979–81 average (3).

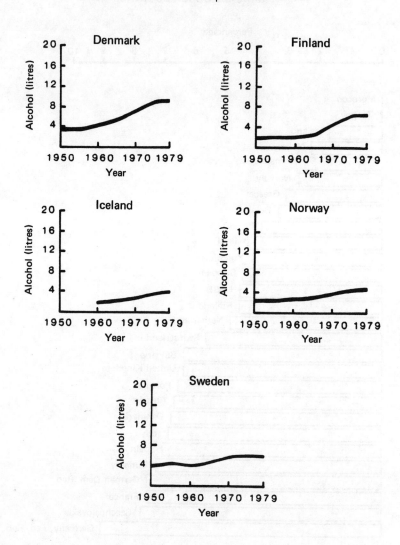

Fig. 46. Consumption of litres of pure alcohol
per head per year
in five northern European countries

Source: Drevon, C.R. (personal communication).

130

7

Formulating nutrition policy objectives: intermediate and ultimate goals

As policy-makers develop proposals to improve the health of a community, opposition may arise once the agriculture and food industries recognize the need to adjust their husbandry, manufacturing and marketing practices. In addition, pressure to change food availability may come from consumers who respond to health education by altering their food purchasing habits or from new government regulations. Governments must necessarily take account of the economic consequences of any proposed changes, but often the cost can be minimized if such changes are specific and then introduced over a reasonable length of time. For example, in Scandinavian and other northern European countries, agricultural production can adapt if the farming industry is encouraged to produce low-fat dairy products and lean meat. Modern production and processing systems can develop products with a much reduced fat content, and encouraging the use of such technology could harness industrial interests to the new health policies.

Fig. 47 shows the nutrient patterns in Europe in relation to both intermediate and ultimate nutrient goals. Four countries have been chosen to illustrate not only the variety of nutrient intake, but also the way in which secular trends are, in general, inappropriate for current needs. For example, there is a worrying increase in saturated fat intake in Italy; this is also seen in Poland. Since the Second World War, Great Britain has experienced a decline in total carbohydrate intake, particularly starch, and a substantial increase in sugar intake. Similarly, Norway has increased its intake of total and of saturated fat.

The dietary patterns of northern Europe are so far from the ideal goals for the prevention of heart disease and high blood pressure that an intermediate policy is needed for any practicable adjustments to be made. Fig. 47 therefore shows intermediate goals that incorporate the recent British and Swedish recommendations. This illustrates the major demands that are going to be made on the makers of policies on health, agriculture and food in the coming years if the burden of ill health is to be reduced. Fig. 38 has already demonstrated how few countries conform even to the intermediate goal for fat consumption developed by national and WHO committees.

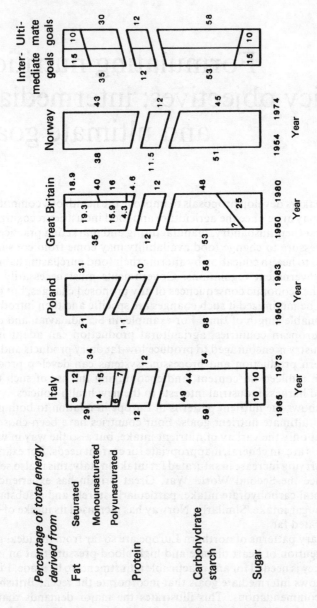

Fig. 47. Nutrient patterns in Europe in relation to intermediate and ultimate goals

Note. Values placed outside the columns are totals; when these can be subdivided the figures are given inside the columns.

Practical Aspects of Policy Implementation

Developing clear terminology is often helpful in dealing with policy issues. This book has so far considered the nutrition objectives developed by WHO committees and groups and national groups of experts. They increasingly use nutrient goals to specify the average optimum intakes of nutrients for the population's health. The term intermediate goal indicates a step towards an ultimate goal. These intermediate goals seem to be required in some countries, where the average nutrient intake is far removed from the ultimate goal and where rapid dietary change could lead to substantial economic and social problems. Ultimate goals are final objectives that may require 20 years or more to achieve.

A food policy is different from a nutrition policy; all countries have a policy on food even if they have none on nutrition. A food policy is the outcome of legislation and government decisions aimed at securing the provision of food for the population, and it incorporates a wide range of measures for fiscal, trading, political, social or consumer protection reasons. A food policy does not necessarily include any explicit consideration of health other than ensuring that sufficient food is available in a form that is safe, or free from microbiological contamination or toxic effects.

Some food policies include explicit nutritional considerations by consciously integrating health issues into their formulation. Governments with this type of policy need to recognize the effects on nutrition and health of possible changes in legislation, taxes or other fiscal or trading measures. This will allow a food policy to be a positive contribution to health rather than simply a reflection of many decisions that exclude any health issue other than the most elementary features of food safety.

A Strategy for Implementing a Nutrition-based Food Policy

The use of the word strategy presupposes that a variety of mechanisms can be identified to help ensure the success of a nutrition-based food policy. Of course, different national needs, opportunities and constraints are likely to lead to many different strategies for implementing policy. It is not for an international agency such as WHO to produce a single organizational model for facilitating progress towards nutrient goals. WHO can contribute, however, by identifying the common themes in existing recommendations, so that nutritional considerations can be formulated into clear policy objectives and be incorporated at an early stage in a more coherent food policy. An analysis of how European countries cope with this problem has not yet been undertaken but will be made in the near future.

Government initiatives, the measures that have an impact on people's diet, can be roughly classified into three categories:

— measures that affect the availability of food to the consumer;

— measures that affect the impact on health of foods; and

— measures that enhance people's knowledge and awareness of food and health issues.

133

Food availability

Some existing legislative and pricing policies in Europe affect the nutrition and health of the European community. An examination of the factors that determine people's choice of foods may reveal that the the cost of individual foods has a large part in determining patterns of food purchases and consumption. For example, existing laws, subsidies or taxes may tend to promote the sale of commodities that would not now be construed as nutritionally important items of the diet. Thus, any measure that tends to reduce the price of sugar, salt or fats and oils with a high content of saturated fat is likely to be disadvantageous. Adjustments in legislation to reduce the price advantages of some commodities could benefit health substantially.

In contrast, some governments may develop specific pricing policies to encourage the consumer to move towards a different pattern of eating. Swedish experts have recently advocated this approach because they consider problems in their country to be serious enough to warrant a major new effort by the central government. Other governments, with a different philosophy, would contend that public education is the best way of achieving change.

The impact of some commodities on health

Many countries already have legislation to control the quality and nature of a variety of food products. Food quality standards are common and are often based not only on the maintenance of standards for food composition traditionally associated with a quality product but also on nutritional criteria. In view of the recent change of emphasis in nutritional thinking described in this book, governments may wish to reassess their legislation on food standards.

Other laws on food have immediate relevance to nutrition. These include, for example, regulations that demand rigorous control of the nutrient composition of substitutes for breast-milk. Food is fortified to ensure an adequate intake of minerals and vitamins in many countries; this can form an important part of any nutritional strategy. In some countries bread is fortified with iron, calcium or vitamins; margarine and milk products may be fortified with fat-soluble vitamins and salt with iodine. The pervasiveness of these regulations reflects governments' concern to ensure the people's welfare, and willingness to legislate on and develop aspects of food policy for health reasons. In most countries, therefore, the tradition is for government to make a positive contribution to improving the nutritional state of the population and not simply to rely on education.

Educating the public

Nutrition education is traditionally seen as involving schools or the media in some form of public health campaign. Nutrition education, however, must permeate the community, and, if change is to occur within the foreseeable future, it must involve the producers and manufacturers of food and policy-makers (politicians and government officials), as well as the public at large. This may require a new approach to education that governments can stimulate. As part of such an approach, food must be labelled to aid consumer choice. The format for labelling, however, requires a great deal of thought. It cannot be geared simply to legislative and regulatory requirements; nutrient labelling must be understood by the average consumer.

A distinction is often made between central policy-making and educating the public. The second approach allows individual choice to determine the national pattern of eating and thereby the economic consequences of a change in demand on food production. Evidence is already accumulating that health education can change consumers' purchasing and eating habits, and major changes are envisaged in some countries as the food and agriculture industries respond to this demand. With foresight, however, these changes can often be handled without major costs to the industries concerned. Health educators can also benefit from working with industrialists, to help in an organized change of policy. Thus, for example, a policy of producing lean meat could, if implemented rapidly, be used to maintain one sector of an industry, such as the production of beef, pork, lamb or mutton, with health educators combining with industry and government to promote the purchase of lean meat. In the absence of readily available lean carcases, however, health educators have little choice but to promote the consumption of poultry, fish and vegetarian food as alternatives. The choice of a collaborative approach, rather than simply expecting industry to respond to consumer demand, may eventually produce major differences in a country's agricultural structure and possibly in its food import and export costs. On this basis alone, some central coordination of a food and health policy would seem sensible.

Educating the public is far from a simple problem and should involve very different groups of people and educational systems. Single public health campaigns are comparatively ineffective; a wide variety of educational approaches is needed.

School curricula

School curricula are likely to be very out of date in their assessment of the role of diet in health; many concepts may be wrong and counterproductive. School curricula may therefore need extensive revision, care being taken to ensure that matters of lifestyle are not seen simply in the context of courses on cookery or biology. A programme aimed at reducing the alarming rate of smoking among teenagers is also to be welcomed.

Health education

Many countries use a centralized information system to inform and educate the public. Often a special section is devoted exclusively to health and its promotion. A separate health education section has advantages in that its relative independence from the central government information system may help convince consumers that educational material is provided for their own good and not for reasons of government finance or other policies.

Health educators commonly believe that simple information is the only requirement for success. In practice, a coherent food and educational policy must evolve in response to a continuous process of reassessing and testing the educational process. Monitoring the effects of education is important because otherwise it is easy to persist with messages that prove to be

135

inappropriate because the citizen puts a different interpretation on them than expected. The educator can also fail to recognize important constraints on changes in lifestyles. Health education should therefore be seen as a progressive process that develops new approaches based on monitored responses and attitudes within the population.

The complex network for the transfer of information and attitudes relating to health needs to be recognized. Community leaders must be involved in any changes. Once the principal messages have permeated the community, local activities can be more important than government policies in determining changes in the sale and production of foods. This is the "bottom up" approach to changes in lifestyle, rather than the "top down" strategy based on central planning.

The role of the media

Newspapers and radio have a large part to play in the educative process, but too often physicians and other professionals engaged in public health avoid contact with the press, radio and television because of fears that their views will be distorted, oversimplified or caricatured to make a subject interesting and controversial. By failing to talk with journalists and commentators, the professionals allow less qualified people to present individual views that often add to people's confusion. The subjects of food and health are intensely interesting to people in all societies, who have recognized the link between the two. The incessant demand for broadcasting material and magazine articles opens a substantial opportunity to change people's perception of nutritious food, but it requires persistence and the willingness of professionals to contribute on many occasions. Some countries have advocated and formed a central clearing agency to which journalists can refer when they want specific information on matters of health.

Health services

Physicians and their colleagues on health care teams are often in an advantageous position to provide an impetus to preventive medicine, but in many countries the teams have become almost exclusively concerned with the management of disease. An effective preventive policy based on primary care is widely regarded as important.

The health services at regional or district level also have many opportunities to develop sound preventive policies. It is possible, for example, to develop a consistent approach to diet in a hospital by involving the catering and dietetic services. This is important for staff, as well as patients. It should be remembered that the health services have, like other government departments, substantial power to adjust the purchasing policies of those who cater for people in the public sector. Regional and district health services lacking a preventive policy should develop one in association with communities. Local industry, trade unions, local shopkeepers and voluntary organizations are particularly important potential contributors.

In all these endeavours, it is now recognized that pursuing an agreed set of objectives with general goodwill is not enough. A regional management plan may be needed, with specific intermediate goals set to test the effectiveness of the drive to improve prevention. Surveys will be needed to establish, for example, how many children and adults in the population still smoke, the proportion of people who have their blood pressure assessed at regular intervals, the types of foods being purchased, and, perhaps, an assessment of the average cholesterol of a subset of the population or the average 24-hour urinary sodium excretion as an index of prevailing salt consumption. An example of a goal-setting policy based on some of the above criteria, with the aim of implementing specific changes within a defined five-year period, was described in the report of the Canterbury Conference *(200)*.

Organizational Structures for the Implementation of a Nutrition Policy

Some of the proposed measures for implementing a nutrition policy will have a substantial impact on the economy and demand very careful planning. Many governments will therefore have to take some overall view of food policy. A group of British experts *(200)* recently advocated the formation of a central government committee to draw on expertise in government departments of economics, trade and industry, agriculture, education, maritime affairs and public information, as well as health. It is hoped that such a committee would evolve a coherent policy that takes into account many of the national issues involved in formulating a food policy. In France, a National Food Council was formed in November 1985 to define a national food policy, to provide guidelines on how to adapt consumption to nutrient requirements, and to consider matters of food safety, food quality and consumer information. In addition to all the government departments concerned with food, the French Government has included national research interests in view of the great need for further research into nutritional aspects of health. The new French Council is under the aegis of the Ministry of Agriculture.

The French approach is likely to allow more readily the recognition of the importance of economic and marketing policies and the way in which current agricultural policies can be adjusted. Some governments may seek to develop pricing policies, including taxes and subsidies, aimed at promoting the consumption of some foods; others may prefer to see more emphasis on the free market economy. Despite the variety of philosophical outlooks and economic management systems employed in the countries of the European Region, however, economic structures already have a substantial effect on people's nutrition.

References

1. *Targets for health for all.* Copenhagen, WHO Regional Office for Europe, 1985, p. 64.
2. **Mason, J.O. & Powell, K.E.** Physical activity, behavioral epidemiology and public health. *Public health reports,* **100**(2): 113–115 (1985).
3. *Food balance sheets, 1979–81 average.* Rome, Food and Agricultural Organization of the United Nations, 1984.
4. *Selected demographic indicators 1950–2000.* New York, United Nations, 1980.
5. **Committee on Medical Aspects of Food Policy, Department of Health and Social Security.** *Diet and cardiovascular disease.* London, H.M. Stationery Office, 1984 (Report on Health and Social Subjects, No. 28).
6. **Cooper, R.** Rising death rates in the Soviet Union. The impact of coronary heart diease. *New England journal of medicine,* **304**: 1259–1265 (1981).
7. **Pisa, Z. & Uemura, K.** Trends of mortality from ischaemic heart disease and other cardiovascular diseases in 27 countries, 1968–1977. *World health statistics quarterly,* **35**(1): 11 (1982).
8. **Pyorala, K. et al.** Trends in coronary heart disease mortality and morbidity and related factors in Finland. *Cardiology,* **72**: 35–51 (1985).
9. *Myocardial infarction community registers.* Copenhagen, WHO Regional Office for Europe, 1976 (Public Health in Europe, No. 5).
10. **Lamm, G.** *The cardiovascular disease programme of WHO in Europe.* Copenhagen, WHO Regional Office for Europe, 1981 (Public Health in Europe, No. 15).
11. **Aho, K. et al.** Cerebrovascular disease in the community: results of a WHO collaborative study. *Bulletin of the World Health Organization,* **58**(1): 113–130 (1980).
12. WHO Technical Report Series, No. 686, 1983 (*Primary prevention of essential hypertension:* report of a WHO Scientific Group).
13. WHO Technical Report Series, No. 727, 1985 (*Diabetes mellitus:* report of a WHO Study Group).
14. **Peto, R. et al.** Can dietary beta-carotene materially reduce human cancer rates? *Nature,* **290**: 201–208 (1981).

15. **Cook-Mozaffari, P.** The epidemiology of cancer of the oesophagus. *Nutrition and cancer,* **1**(2): 51–59 (1979).
16. **Napalkov, N.P. et al., ed.** *Cancer incidence in the USSR.* Lyon, International Agency for Research on Cancer, 1982 (IARC Scientific Publications, No. 48).
17. **Tulinius, H.** Epidemiology of gastric cancer. *Nutrition and cancer,* **1**: 61–69 (1979).
18. **Wynder, E.L. et al.** Nutrition and metabolic epidemiology of cancers of the oral cavity, oesophagus, colon, breast, prostate and stomach. *In:* Newell, G.R. & Ellison, N.M., ed. *Nutrition and cancer: etiology and treatment.* New York, Raven Press, 1981.
19. **Jensen, O.M.** Cancer of the large bowel: a three-fold variation between Denmark and Finland. *Nutrition and cancer,* **4**(1): 20–22 (1982).
20. **Waterhouse, J. et al.** *Cancer incidence in five continents.* Lyon, International Agency for Research on Cancer, 1976, Vol. 3 (IARC Scientific Publications, No. 15).
21. La mortalità in Italia, 1970–79 [Mortality in Italy, 1970–79]. *Rapporti Istisan,* June 1984.
22. **Walsh, D.** *Alcohol-related medicosocial problems and their prevention.* Copenhagen, WHO Regional Office for Europe, 1982 (Public Health in Europe, No. 17).
23. **Silberberg, R.** Obesity and osteoarthrosis. *In:* Mancini, M. et al., ed. *Medical complications of obesity.* London, Academic Press, 1979, pp. 301–315.
24. **Engel, A.** Osteoarthritis and body measurements. *Vital health statistics,* **11**: 1–37 (1968).
25. **Mannius, S. et al.** The incidence of hip fractures in a large city and in a rural district in Sweden. *In:* Dehlin, O. & Stein, B., ed. *Second Nordic Congress on Gerontology.* Täby, Santos, 1984, pp. 289–291.
26. **Boyce, W.J. & Vessey, M.P.** Rising incidence of fracture of proximal femur. *Lancet,* **1**: 150–151 (1985).
27. **Nilsson, B.E. & Obrant, K.J.** Secular tendencies of the incidence of fracture of the upper end of the femur. *Acta orthopaedica Scandinavica,* **49**: 389–391 (1978).
28. **Sreebny, L.M.** Sugar availability, sugar consumption and dental caries. *Community dentistry and oral epidemiology,* **10**: 1–7 (1982).
29. WHO Technical Report Series, No. 405, 1968 (*Nutritional anaemias: report of a WHO Scientific Group*).
30. **Rybo, E.** Diagnosis of iron deficiency. *Scandinavian journal of haematology,* **34**(Suppl. No. 43) (1985).
31. **Bengtsson, C. et al.** Prevalence and reasons for anaemia in a population sample in Gothenburg, Sweden, in 1968–69, 1974–75 and 1980–81. *Colloque INSERM/ISTA,* **113**: 14–48 (1983).
32. **Damberg, S.E.** Prevalence of anaemia in Denmark. *In:* Hallberg, L. & Solvell, L., ed. *Iron deficiency and iron therapy.* Gothenburg, AB Hassle, 1978, pp. 144–148.

33. **Hagerup, L. et al.** The Glostrup population studies. Collection of epidemiologic tables. *Scandinavian journal of social medicine,* **20**: 1–112 (1981).

34. **Milman, N. et al.** Iron stores in female blood donors evaluated by serum ferritin. *Blut,* **51**(5): 337–345 (1985).

35. **Vellar, D.D.** Iron deficiency in adults in Norway. *In:* Hallberg, L. & Solvell, L., ed. *Iron deficiency and iron therapy.* Gothenburg, AB Hassle, 1978, pp. 128–135.

36. **Elwood, P.C. et al.** An international haematological survey. *Bulletin of the World Health Organization,* **54**: 87–95 (1976).

37. **Takkunen, H.** Iron deficiency in the Finnish adult population. An epidemiological survey from 1967 to 1972 inclusive. *Scandinavian journal of haematology,* Suppl. No. 25 (1976).

38. **Galan, P. et al.** Factors affecting iron stores in French female students. *Human nutrition: clinical nutrition,* **39C**: 279–287 (1985).

39. **Arab, L. et al.** Nutrition and health. A survey of young men and women in Heidelberg. *Annals of nutrition and metabolism,* **26**(Suppl. No. 1): 1–224 (1982).

40. **Saliev, K.K. et al.** Primenenie polifunktsional'nogo krovezamenitelia polifora dlia lecheniia bol'nykh zhelezodefitsitnoj anemiej [Multifunctional blood substitute in the treatment of iron-deficiency anaemia]. *Gematologiia transfuziologiia,* **28**(6): 14–16 (1983).

41. **Taylor, D.J. & Lind, T.** Haematological changes during normal pregnancy: iron induced macrocytosis. *British journal of obstetrics and gynaecology,* **83**: 760 (1976).

42. **Hytten, F.E. & Lind, T.** *Diagnostic indices in pregnancies.* Basle, Ciba Geigy, 1973.

43. **Taylor, D.J. et al.** The effect of oral supplementation upon serum ferritin levels during and after pregnancy. *British journal of obstetrics and gynaecology,* **89**: 1011 (1982).

44. **Marshavelova, Y. et al.** Iron deficiency in children aged 1–3 years. *Folia medica,* **21**(1): 48–50 (1979).

45. **Ziemlanski, S. & Charzewska, J.** Nutritional anaemia in selected groups of children and youth of Warsaw and Ciechanow schools. *Acta medica Polona,* **19**(4): 468–477 (1978).

46. **Schuler, D. et al.** Vashiány és vaspótlás a csecsemökorban [Iron deficiency and iron substitution in infancy]. *Orvosi hetilap,* **123**(2): 91–93 (1982).

47. **Borgstrom, B. et al., ed.** Nutrition and old age. *Scandinavian journal of gastroenterology,* **14**(Suppl. No. 52) (1979).

48. **Department of Health and Social Security.** *Nutrition and health in old age.* London, H.M. Stationery Office, 1979 (Report on Health and Social Subjects, No. 16).

49. **Durand, H. et al.** Fréquence et étiologie des anémies chez les personnes âgées de plus de 70 ans [Frequency and etiology of anaemias in elderly people aged over 70 years]. *Semaine des hôpitaux de Paris,* **55**: 1782–1787 (1979).

50. **Smithells, R.W.** Diet and congenital malformation. *In:* Campbell, D.M. & Gillmer, M.D.G. *Nutrition in pregnancy.* London, Royal College of Obstetricians and Gynaecologists, 1983, pp. 155–165.

51. **Lawrence, K.M. et al.** Increased risk of recurrence of pregnancies complicated by foetal neural tube defects in mothers receiving poor diets, and possible benefit of dietary counselling. *British medical journal,* **281**: 1592–1594 (1980).

52. **Subcommittee for the Study of Endemic Goitre and Iodine Deficiency of the European Thyroid Association.** Goitre and iodine deficiency in Europe. *Lancet,* **1**: 1289–1293 (1985).

53. **Hetzel, B.S.** Iodine deficiency disorders (IDD) and their eradication. *Lancet,* **2**: 1126–1129 (1983).

54. **Bender, A.E. & Brookes, L.J., ed.** *Body weight control. Proceedings of the First International Meeting on Body Weight Control, Montreux, Switzerland, April 1985.* London, Churchill Livingston, 1987.

55. **Bray, G.A., ed.** Obesity in perspective. *Proceedings of the 2nd Fogarty International Centre Conference on Obesity.* Washington, DC, US Department of Health, Education and Welfare, 1975 (Publication No. (NIH) 75-708).

56. Obesity: a report of the Royal College of Physicians, London. *Journal of the Royal College of Physicians,* **17**(1) (1983).

57. **Garrow, J.S.** *Treat obesity seriously. A clinical manual.* London, Churchill Livingston, 1981.

58. **Kluthe, R. & Schubert, A.** Obesity in Europe. *Annals of internal medicine,* **103**: 1037–1042 (1985).

59. **Mancini, M. et al.** Medical complications and prevalence of obesity in Italy. *In:* Somogyi, J.L. & Trichopoulou, A. *Scientific evidence for dietary targets in Europe,* Basle, Karger, 1986, pp. 1–10 (Bibliotheca Nutritio et Dieta, No. 37).

60. **Knight, I.** *Heights and weights of adults in Great Britain.* London, H.M. Stationery Office, 1984.

61. **Waaler, H.T.** Height, weight and mortality: the Norwegian experience. *Acta medica Scandinavica* (Suppl. No. 679) (1984).

62. **Garrow, J.S.** Indices of adiposity. *Nutrition abstracts and reviews, series A,* **53**(8): 697–708 (1983).

63. **Society of Actuaries.** *Build study 1979.* Chicago, Society of Actuaries and Association of Life Insurance Medical Directors, 1979.

64. **Lew, E.A. & Garfinkel, L.** Variations in mortality by weight among 750 000 men and women. *Journal of chronic disorders,* **32**: 563–576 (1979).

65. **James, W.P.T.** Treatment of obesity: the constraints on success. *In: Clinics in epidemiology.* London, W.B. Saunders, 1984, Vol. 13, pp. 635–659.

66. **Larsson, B. et al.** Abdominal adipose tissue distribution, obesity, and risk of cardiovascular disease and death: 13-year follow-up of participants in the study of men born in 1913. *British medical journal,* **288**: 1401–1404 (1984).

67. **Kesteloot, H. & Van Houte, O.** An epidemiological survey of arterial blood pressure in a large male population group. *American journal of epidemiology,* **99**: 14–29 (1974).

68. **Kannel, W.B.** An overview of the risk factors for cardiovascular disease. *In:* Kaplan, N.M. & Stamler, J., ed. *Prevention of coronary heart disease — practical management of the risk factors.* Philadelphia, PA, W.B. Saunders, 1983.

69. **Cox, H. & Marks, L.** Sales trends and survey findings: a study of smoking in 15 OECD countries. *Health trends,* **15**: 48–51 (1983).

70. **Keys, A.** *Seven countries: a multivariate analysis of death and coronary heart disease.* London, Harvard University Press, 1980.

71. **Ross, R. & Glomset, J.A.** The pathogenesis of atherosclerosis. *New England journal of medicine,* **295**(8): 420–425 (1976).

72. **Ross, R.** Pathogenesis of atherosclerosis — an update. *New England journal of medicine,* **314**: 488–500 (1986).

73. **Keys, A. et al.** Serum cholesterol response to changes in the diet. III. Differences among individuals. *Metabolism,* **14**: 766–775 (1965).

74. **Hegstead, D.M. et al.** Quantitative effects of dietary fat on serum cholesterol in man. *American journal of clinical nutrition,* **17**: 281–293 (1965).

75. **Morris, J.N. et al.** Diet and heart: a postscript. *British medical journal,* **2**: 1307–1314 (1977).

76. **Kushi, L.H. et al.** Diet and 20-year mortality from coronary heart disease. The Ireland-Boston diet-heart study. *New England journal of medicine,* **312**(13): 811–818 (1985).

77. **Welin, L. et al.** Why is the incidence of ischaemic heart disease in Sweden increasing? Study of men born in 1913 and 1923. *Lancet,* **1**: 1087–1089 (1983).

78. **Isaksson, B.** A report on the nutrition policy in Sweden. Beltsville Symposium in Agricultural Research, No. 4. *In:* Beecher, G.R., ed. *Human nutrition research.* Toronto, Allanheld, Osmun & Co., 1981, pp. 259–270.

79. **Rouse, I.L. et al.** Blood-pressure-lowering effects of a vegetarian diet: controlled trial in normotensive subjects. *Lancet,* **1**: 5–10 (1983).

80. **Arntzenius, A.C. et al.** Diet, lipoproteins, and the progression of coronary atherosclerosis. The Leiden intervention trial. *New England journal of medicine,* **312**(13): 805–811 (1985).

81. **Miller, G.J. & Miller, N.E.** Plasma-high-density-lipoprotein concentration and development of ischaemic heart-disease. *Lancet,* **1**: 16–19 (1975).

82. **Thelle, S. et al.** British heart study. *British heart journal,* **49**: 205 (1983).

83. **Hjermann, I. et al.** Effect of diet and smoking intervention on the incidence of coronary heart disease. *Lancet,* **2**: 1303–1310 (1981).

84. **Multiple Risk Factor Intervention Trial Research Group.** Multiple Risk Factor Intervention Trial — risk factor changes and mortality results. *Journal of the American Medical Association,* **248**: 1464–1477 (1982).

85. **Lipid Research Clinics.** Coronary primary prevention trial results. 1. Reduction in incidence of coronary heart disease. *Journal of the American Medical Association,* **251**(3): 351–374 (1984).

86. **WHO European Collaborative Group.** Multifactorial trial in the prevention of coronary heart disease. 3. Incidence and mortality results. *European heart journal,* **4**: 141–147 (1983).

87. **WHO European Collaborative Group.** European collaborative trial of multifactorial prevention of coronary heart disease: final report on the 6-year results. *Lancet,* **1**: 869–872 (1986).

88. **Puska, P. et al.** The community-based strategy to prevent coronary heart disease: conclusions from the ten years of the North Karelia Project. *Annual review of public health,* **6**: 147–193 (1985).

89. **Goldman, L. & Cook, E.F.** The decline in ischaemic heart disease mortality rates: an analysis of the comparative effects of medical interventions and changes in lifestyle. *Annals of internal medicine,* **101**: 825–836 (1984).

90. **Norum, K.R.** Ways and means of influencing national nutritional behaviour. Experience from the Norwegian nutrition and food policy. *In: Influence of modern style of life on food habits of man.* Basle, Karger, 1985, pp. 29–43 (Bibliotheca Nutritio et Dieta, No. 36).

91. **Isaksson, B.** Diet and exercise: assessment of the Swedish programme. A Swedish approach to nutrition in obesity. *In:* Bray, G., ed. *Recent advances in obesity research. II. Proceedings of the 2nd International Congress on Obesity.* London, Newman Publishing, 1978, pp. 477–485.

92. **Kelly, A. & Kevany, J.** *Nutritional surveillance in Ireland: report for 1984.* Dublin, Medico-Social Research Board for Ireland, 1985.

93. **Brown, J.J. et al.** Salt and hypertension. Letter. *Lancet,* **2**: 456 (1984).

94. WHO Technical Report Series, No. 678, 1982 (*Prevention of coronary heart disease:* report of a WHO Expert Committee).

95. **Gleiberman, L.** Blood pressure and dietary salt in human populations. *Ecology of food and nutrition,* **2**: 143–156 (1973).

96. **McCarron, D.A.** Calcium and magnesium nutrition in human hypertension. *Annals of internal medicine,* **98**: 800–805 (1983).

97. **Lever, A.F. et al.** Sodium and potassium in essential hypertension. *British medical journal,* **283**: 463–468 (1981).

98. **Meneely, G.R. et al.** Chronic sodium toxicity: the protective effect of added potassium chloride. *Annals of internal medicine,* **47**: 263–273 (1957).

99. **MacGregor, G.A. et al.** Moderate potassium supplementation in essential hypertension. *Lancet,* **2**: 567–570 (1982).

100. **Kotchen, T.A. et al.** Effect of chloride on renin and blood pressure responses to sodium chloride. *Annals of internal medicine,* **98**: 817–822 (1983).

101. **Puska, P. et al.** Controlled randomised trial of dietary fat on blood pressure. *Lancet,* **1**: 1–4 (1983).

102. **Iacono, J.M. et al.** Reduction of blood pressure associated with dietary polyunsaturated fat. *Hypertension,* **4**(Suppl. No. III): 34–42 (1982).

103. **Huttunen, J.K. et al.** Dietary factors and hypertension. *Acta medica Scandinavica,* (Suppl. No. 701): 72–82 (1985).
104. **MacGregor, G.A.** Double-blind randomised crossover trial of moderate potassium restriction in essential hypertension. *Lancet,* **1**: 351–355 (1982).
105. **Parijs, J. et al.** Moderate sodium restriction and diuretics in the treatment of hypertension. *American heart journal,* **85**: 22–34 (1973).
106. **Morgan, T. et al.** Hypertension treated with salt restriction. *Lancet,* **1**: 227–230 (1978).
107. **Magnani, B. et al.** Comparison of the effects of pharmacological therapy and a low-sodium diet on mild hypertension. *Clinical science,* **51**: 625s–626s (1976).
108. **Holly, J.M.P. et al.** Reanalysis of data in two *Lancet* papers on the effect of dietary sodium and potassium on blood pressure. *Lancet,* **2**: 1384–1387 (1982).
109. **Beard, T.C. et al.** Randomised controlled trial of a no-added-sodium diet for mild hypertension. *Lancet,* **2**: 455–458 (1982).
110. **Watt, G.M.C. et al.** Dietary sodium restriction for mild hypertension in general practice. *British medical journal,* **286**: 432–436 (1983).
111. **Gillum, R.F. et al.** Changing sodium intake in children: the Minneapolis children's blood pressure study. *Hypertension,* **3**: 698–703 (1981).
112. **Richards, A.M. et al.** Blood pressure response to moderate sodium restriction and to potassium supplementation in mild essential hypertension. *Lancet,* **1**: 757–761 (1984).
113. **Joossens, J.V. & Geboers, J.** Salt and hypertension. *Preventive medicine,* **12**: 53–59 (1983).
114. **Helgarson, T. et al.** Diabetes produced in mice by smoked/cured mutton. *Lancet,* **2**: 1017–1022 (1982).
115. **Doll, R. & Peto, R.** *Causes of cancer.* Oxford, Oxford Medical Publications, 1981.
116. **King, M.M. et al.** Dietary fat may influence DMBA-mediated mammary gland carcinogenesis by modification of mammary gland development. *In:* Roe, D.A., ed. *Diet, nutrition and cancer: from basic research to policy implications.* New York, Alan Liss, 1983, pp. 61–90 (Current Topics in Nutrition and Disease, Vol. 9).
117. **Committee on Diet, Nutrition, and Cancer. Assembly of Life Sciences. National Research Council.** *Diet, nutrition, and cancer.* Washington, DC, National Academy Press, 1982.
118. *Cancer. Orsaker, förebyggande, mm. Betänkande av Cancerkommitten* [Cancer. Causes, prevention, etc. Report of the Cancer Committee]. Stockholm, Socialdepartmentet, 1984 (Statens Offentliga Utredningar, No. 67).
119. **Joossens, J.V. et al., ed.** *Diet and human carcinogenesis. Proceedings of the 3rd ECP Symposium, 19–21 June 1985, Aarhus, Denmark.* London, Elsevier, 1986 (International Congress Series, No. 685).
120. **Tuyns, A. et al.** Le cancer de l'œsophage en Ille-et-Vilaine en fonction des niveaux de consommation d'alcool et de tabac [Cancer of the

oesophagus in Ille-et-Vilaine in relation to levels of consumption of alcohol and tobacco]. *Bulletin du cancer,* **64**(1): 45–60 (1977).

121. **Joossens, J.V.** Stroke, stomach cancer and salt: a possible clue to the prevention of hypertension. *In:* Kesteloot, H. & Joossens, J.V., ed. *Epidemiology of arterial blood pressure. Developments in cardiovascular medicine.* The Hague, Martinus Nijhoff, 1980, pp. 489–508.

122. **Trichopoulos, D. et al.** Diet and cancer of the stomach: a case-control study in Greece. *International journal of cancer,* **36**: 291–297 (1985).

123. **Armstrong, B. & Doll, R.** Environmental factors and cancer incidence and mortality in different countries with special reference to dietary practices. *International journal of cancer,* **15**: 617–631 (1975).

124. **Burkitt, D.P.** Epidemiology of cancer of the colon and rectum. *Cancer,* **28**: 3–31 (1971).

125. **Cummings, J.** Cancer of the large bowel. *In:* Trowell, H. et al., ed. *Dietary fibre, fibre-depleted foods and disease.* London, Academic Press, 1985, pp. 161–189.

126. **McMichael, A.J. et al.** Time trends in colorectal cancer mortality in relation to food and alcohol consumption: United States, United Kingdom, Australia and New Zealand. *International journal of epidemiology,* **8**(4): 295–303 (1979).

127. **Muir, C.S. & James, P.** Diet and large bowel cancer in Denmark and Finland: report of the Second IARC International Collaborative Study. *Nutrition and cancer,* **4**: 1–79 (1982).

128. **Heaton, K.W.** The role of diet in the etiology of colilithiasis. *Nutrition abstracts and reviews, series A,* **54**: 549–560 (1984).

129. **Parfitt, A.M.** Dietary risk factors for age-related bone loss and fractures. *Lancet,* **2**: 1181–1184 (1983).

130. **Nordin, B.E.C. et al.** Calcium requirement and calcium therapy. *Clinical orthopaedics,* **140**: 216–239 (1979).

131. **Markovic, V. et al.** Bone status and fracture rates in two regions of Yugoslavia. *American journal of clinical nutrition,* **32**: 540–549 (1979).

132. **Parfitt, A.M. et al.** Vitamin D and bone health in the elderly. *American journal of clinical nutrition,* **36**: 1014–1031 (1982).

133. **Yuen, D.E. et al.** Effect of dietary protein on calcium metabolism in man. *Nutrition abstracts and reviews, series A,* **54**: 447–459 (1984).

134. **Bernstein, D.S. et al.** Prevalence of osteoporosis in high- and low-fluoride areas in North Dakota. *Journal of the American Medical Association,* **198**: 499–504 (1966).

135. **Riggs, B.L. et al.** Effect of the fluoride/calcium regimen on vertebral fracture occurrence in post-menopausal osteoporosis. *New England journal of medicine,* **306**(8): 446–450 (1982).

136. **Sheiham, A.** Sugars and dental decay. *Lancet,* **1**: 282–284 (1983).

137. **Takeuchi, D.D.S.** Epidemiological study on dental caries in Japanese children before, during and after World War II. *International dental journal,* **11**: 443–457 (1961).

138. **Schulerud, A.** *Dental caries and nutrition during wartime in Norway.* Oslo, Fabritius & Sønners Trykkeri, 1950.

139. *FAO/WHO joint report. Carbohydrates in human nutrition.* Rome, Food and Agriculture Organization of the United Nations, 1980 (FAO Food and Nutrition Papers, No. 15).

140. **Marthaler, T.M.** Sugar and oral health. *In:* Guggenheim, B.S., ed. *Health and sugar substitutes.* Basle, Karger, 1979.

141. **Burt, B.A. & Ekland, S.A.** Sugar consumption and dental caries. Some epidemiological patterns. *In: US Fourth Annual Conference on Foods, Nutrition and Dental Health.* Chicago, American Dental Association, 1980.

142. **Newbrun, E.** Sugar and dental caries: a review of human studies. *Science,* **217**: 418–423 (1982).

143. **Takeuchi, D.D.S.** Epidemiological study on relation between dental caries incidence and sugar consumption. *Bulletin of Tokyo Dental College,* **1**: 58–70 (1960).

144. **Shimamura, S.** A cohort survey on caries attacks in permanent teeth during a period of approximately 20 kg of annual sugar consumption per person in Japan. *Journal of dental health,* **24**: 46–52 (1974).

145. **Wass, R.L. & Trithart, A.H.** Between-meal eating habits and dental caries experience in preschool children. *American journal of public health,* **50**: 1097 (1960).

146. **Rugg-Gunn, A.J.** Diet and dental caries. *In:* Murray, J.J., ed. *Prevention of dental disease.* Oxford, Oxford University Press, 1983, pp. 3–82.

147. **Sognnaes, R.F.** Analysis of wartime reduction of dental caries in European children. *American journal of diseases of childhood,* **75**: 792 (1948).

148. **British Association for the Study of Community Dentistry.** *Sugar and dental caries: a policy statement.* Manchester, Tameside Health Authority, 1982.

149. **Gustaffson, B.E. et al.** Vipeholm study. *Acta odontologica Scandinavica,* **11**: 232 (1954).

150. **Scheinin, A. & Makinen, K.K.** Turku study. *Acta odontologica Scandinavica,* **33**(Suppl. No. 70) (1975).

151. **King, J.D. et al.** *The effect of sugar supplements on dental caries in children.* London, H.M. Stationery Office, 1955 (British Medical Research Council Special Report No. 288).

152. **von der Fehr, F.R. et al.** Experimental caries in man. *Caries research,* **4**: 131 (1970).

153. **Geddes, D.A.M.L. et al.** *Archives of oral biology,* **23**: 663 (1978).

154. **Bowen, W.H. et al.** A method to assess cariogenic potential of foodstuffs. *Journal of the American Dental Association,* **100**(5): 677–681 (1980).

155. *A summary of the report from the Expert Group for Diet and Health.* Uppsala, Expert Group for Diet and Health, 1985.

156. *On the follow-up of the Norwegian nutrition policy.* Oslo, Ministry of Health and Social affairs, 1982 (Report to the Storting, No. 11).

157. WHO Technical Report Series, No. 713, 1984 (*Prevention methods and programmes for oral diseases:* report of a WHO Expert Committee).

158. **International Programme on Chemical Safety (IPCS).** *Fluorine and fluorides.* Geneva, World Health Organization, 1984 (Environmental Health Criteria, No. 36).

159. **Fédération dentaire internationale.** Goals for oral health in the year 2000. *FDI newsletter,* March (1982).

160. **Hallberg, L. et al.** Low bioavailability of carbonyl iron in man: studies on iron fortification of wheat flour. *American journal of clinical nutrition,* **43**(1): 59–67 (1986).

161. **Herbertsson, M.** The nutritional contents of the food. *Journal of agricultural economics,* **47**(7–8): 293–308 (1985).

162. **Hallberg, L.** Fetma hos kvinnor i olika åldrar. Kaleriintag och födoämnesval [Fat in women at different ages. Calorie intake and choice of foods]. *Läkartidningen,* **63**: 611–626 (1966).

163. **Haraldsdottir, J. et al.** *Danskernes kostvaner 1985* [Danish eating habits 1985]. Copenhagen, Levnedsmiddelstyrelsen, 1985.

164. *Food consumption statistics 1973–82.* Paris, Organisation for Economic Co-operation and Development, 1985.

165. **Wickham, C. et al.** Seasonal variation in folate nutritional status. *Irish journal of medical science,* **152**: 295–299 (1983).

166. **Poh Tan, S. et al.** Folic acid content of the diet in various British households. *Human nutrition: applied nutrition,* **38A**: 17–22 (1984).

167. **Jagerstad, M. et al.** Folates. *Scandinavian journal of social medicine,* 3(Suppl. No. 10): 78–83 (1975).

168. **Jagerstad, M. & Westesson, A.-K.** Folates. *Scandinavian journal of gastroenterology,* **14**(Suppl. No. 52): 196–202 (1979).

169. **Elsborg, L. & Rosenquist, A.** Folate intake by teenage girls and pregnant women. *International journal of vitamin and nutrition research,* **49**: 70–76 (1979).

170. **Hessov, I. & Elsborg, L.** Nutritional studies on long-term surgical patients with special reference to vitamin B12 and folic acid. *International journal of vitamin and nutrition research,* **46**: 427–432 (1983).

171. *FAO/WHO joint report. Dietary fats and oils in human nutrition.* Rome, Food and Agriculture Organization of the United Nations, 1980 (FAO Food and Nutrition Series, No. 20).

172. **Kannel, W.B. & Gordon, T., ed.** *Section 26. Some characteristics related to the incidence of cardiovascular disease and death: Framingham study, 16-year follow-up.* Washington, DC, US Government Printing Office, 1970.

173. **Pooling Project Research Group.** Relationship of blood pressure, serum cholesterol, smoking habit, relative weight and ECG abnormalities to incidence of major coronary events: final report of the Pooling Project. *Journal of chronic diseases,* **31**: 201–306 (1978).

174. **Oliver, M.F.** Serum cholesterol — the knave of hearts and the joker. *Lancet,* **2**: 192–204 (1981).

175. Dutch dietary guidelines. *Voeding,* **47**: 140 (1986).

176. WHO Technical Report Series, No. 732, 1986 (*Community prevention and control of cardiovascular diseases:* report of a WHO Expert Committee).

148

177. **Rose, G.A.** Strategy of prevention: lessons from cardiovascular disease. *British medical journal,* **282**: 1847–1851 (1981).

178. **Wilhelmsen, L. et al.** Salt and hypertension. *Clinical science,* **57**(Suppl. No. 5): 455–458 (1979).

179. **Marmot, M.G.** Diet, hypertension and stroke. *In:* Turner, M.R., ed. *Nutrition and health.* London, MTP Press, 1982, pp. 243–254.

180. **Grimm, R.H., Jr, et al.** Effects of thiazide diuretics on plasma lipids and lipoproteins in mildly hypertensive patients. A double-blind controlled trial. *Annals of internal medicine,* **94**: 7–11 (1981).

181. **Langford, H.G. et al.** Dietary therapy slows the return of hypertension after stopping prolonged medication. *Journal of the American Medical Association,* **253**: 657–664 (1985).

182. **Stamler, R. et al.** Primary prevention of hypertension — a randomized controlled trial. *Annals of clinical research,* **16**(Suppl. No. 43): 136–142 (1984).

183. **Stamler, J. et al.** Prevention and control of hypertension by nutritional-hygienic means. Long-term experiences in the Chicago coronary prevention evaluation program. *Journal of the American Medical Association,* **243**: 1819–1823 (1980).

184. Rationale of the diet–heart statement of the American Heart Association. *Arteriosclerosis,* **4**: 177–191 (1982).

185. **Brody, J.A.** Prospects for an ageing population. *Nature,* **315**: 463–466 (1985).

186. **The US/USSR Steering Committee for Problem Area 1: the Pathogenesis of Atherosclerosis.** Nutrient intake and its association with high-density lipoprotein and low-density lipoprotein cholesterol in selected US and USSR subpopulations. *American journal of clinical nutrition,* **39**: 942–952 (1984).

187. **Ministry of Agriculture, Fisheries and Food.** *Household food consumption and expenditure: annual report of the National Food Survey Committee.* London, H.M. Stationery Office, 1984.

188. **Walker, C.L.** The national diet. *Postgraduate medical journal,* **60**(699): 26–33 (1984).

189. **Ferro-Luzzi, A. & Sette, S.** Changing dietary habits in Italy as related to cardiovascular diseases. *In: New trends in nutrition, lipid research, and cardiovascular diseases.* New York, Alan Liss, 1981, pp. 231–241.

190. **Menotti, A. et al.** Recent trends in coronary heart disease and other cardiovascular diseases in Italy. *Cardiology,* **72**: 88–96 (1985).

191. **Isaksson, B.** Requirements *and* appropriate *intakes of electrolytes.* Basle, Karger, 1983, pp. 42–60 (Bibliotheca Nutritrio et Dieta, No. 33).

192. **Knuiman, J.T. et al.** A multi-centre study on within-person variability in the urinary excretion of sodium, potassium, calcium, magnesium and creatinine in 8 European centres. *Human nutrition: clinical nutrition,* **40**(5): 343–348 (1986).

193. **Pietinen, P.** Estimating sodium intake from food consumption data. *Annals of nutrition metabolism,* **26**: 90–99 (1982).

194. **Seppanen, R. et al.** Summary: the food consumption and nutrient intake in Finland from 1973 to 1976. *Kansaneläkelaitoksen Julkaisuja,* **22**: 133 (1981).
195. **Pietinen, P.** Sources of sodium in the Finnish diet. *Journal of the Scientific Agricultural Society of Finland,* **53**: 275–284 (1981).
196. **Westin, S.** Genomsnittlig konsumtion av natrium och klorid [Average consumption of sodium and chloride]. *Vår föda,* **32**: 321–325 (1980).
197. **Bull, N.L. & Buss, D.H.** Contribution of foods to sodium intake. *Proceedings of the Nutrition Society,* **39**: 30A (1980).
198. **Bowen, R.E. et al.** Proceedings: designing formulated foods for the cardiac-concerned. *Preventive medicine,* **2**: 366–377 (1973).
199. **James, W.P.T. et al.** The dominance of salt in manufactured food in the sodium intake of affluent societies. *Lancet,* **1**: 426–429 (1987).
200. *Coronary heart disease. Plans for action: report of the Canterbury Conference.* London, Pitman, 1984.